TASTY. NAUGHTY. HEALTHY. NICE.

Tasty
Naug
Health

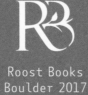

Roost Books
Boulder 2017

Whole Food Made Sinfully Delicious

Susan Jane White

hty.

y · Nice.

Roost Books
An imprint of Shambhala Publications, Inc.
4720 Walnut Street
Boulder, Colorado 80301
roostbooks.com

9 8 7 6 5 4 3 2 1

First U.S. Edition
Printed in China

♾ This edition is printed on acid-free paper that meets the American National
Standards Institute Z39.48 Standard.
♲ Shambhala Publications makes every effort to print on recycled paper.
For more information please visit www.shambhala.com.

Distributed in the United States by Penguin Random House LLC and in Canada by
Random House of Canada Ltd

Library of Congress Cataloging-in-Publication Data

Names: White, Susan Jane, author.
Title: Tasty. Naughty. Healthy. Nice: whole food made sinfully delicious /
Susan Jane White.
Description: First U.S. edition. | Boulder: Roost, 2017. | Includes index.
"Originally published by Gill Books, 2014."
Identifiers: LCCN 2016030394 | ISBN 9781611804362 (hardcover: alk. paper)
Subjects: LCSH: Cooking (Natural foods) | Sugar-free diet–Recipes. |
Wheat-free diet–Recipes. | Milk-free diet–Recipes. | LCGFT: Cookbooks.
Classification: LCC TX741.W464 2017 | DDC 641.3/02–dc23 LC record
available at https://lccn.loc.gov/2016030394

CONTENTS

\+ + + + + + + +

SNACKS AND OTHER NUTRITIONAL HITS

Superfood Spreads

SOUPS

SALADS

Spiralizer Recipes

SUPPERS

TASTY HEALTHY TREATS

WHAT TO READ AND WHERE TO SHOP

INDEX

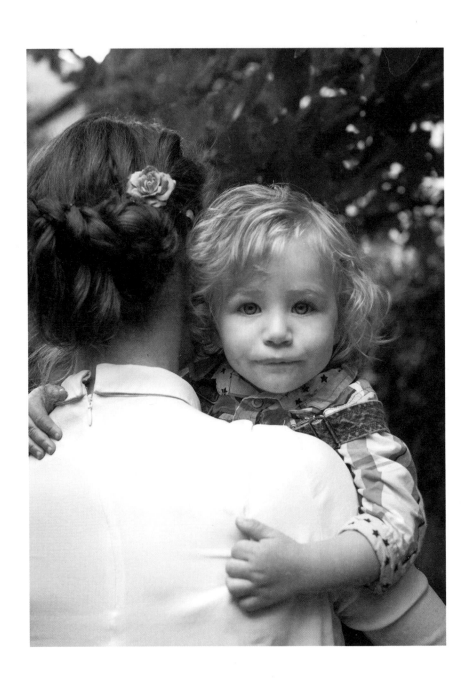

ACKNOWLEDGMENTS

To Sara Bercholz, for skillfully navigating my crazy-Irish-lady vibe.
Thank you for taking a chance on me. To you, I owe so much.

To Jennifer Urban-Brown, my sassy, savvy editor who catapulted my work
into another stratosphere. Without you, I'd still be in the clouds.

A high-five to the wonderful Audra Figgins, my surrogate Irish bro Steven
Pomije, and legendary hustler KJ. You gave this book a Formula One engine.
Thunderous thanks.

To the dazzling team that is Roost Books. I hope you catch my consignment of
love-bombs crossing the Atlantic every week. I think you're magical.

A thunderous thank you to photographer Jo Murphy, stylist Orla Neligan, and
assistants Kerrie and Liosa. I never expected to have so much fun or to make new
friends in the process. Working with you all was beyond inspiring.

Tom Dunne and producer Joe Donnelly—radio was never so much fun.
A heartfelt thank you.

My agent Rebecca Morgan for her tenacity, loyalty, and tireless enthusiasm.
Thank you for putting up with me these past fourteen years.

I'm grateful to Oliver and his team at Wall & Keogh in Portobello,
where I spend hours sipping gorgeous teas, tapping toes, and writing.

To my beloved, the most nourishing superfood my body has ever known.
You electrify me. Mostly.

Our adorable boys, Benjamin and Marty, whose laughter rings through our home.

To mum. What a marvel.

Many impressive commentators and activists continue to inspire and inform me.
My sincere gratitude to you all: Joanna Blythman, Felicity Lawrence,
Bee Wilson, Mark Bittman, Michael Pollan, Marion Nestle, Robyn O'Brien,
Dr. David A. Kessler, Michael Moss, Gary Taubes, Dr Marilyn Glenville,
Eric Schlosser, Robert Lustig, Hugh Fearnley-Whittingstall, Dr John Briffa,
Dr John McKenna, Colin Tudge, Claudia Hammond, and George Monbiot.

And lastly, YOU. I have the best readers in the world.
You give flight to my imagination and make it all possible for me.
I wrote this book for you.

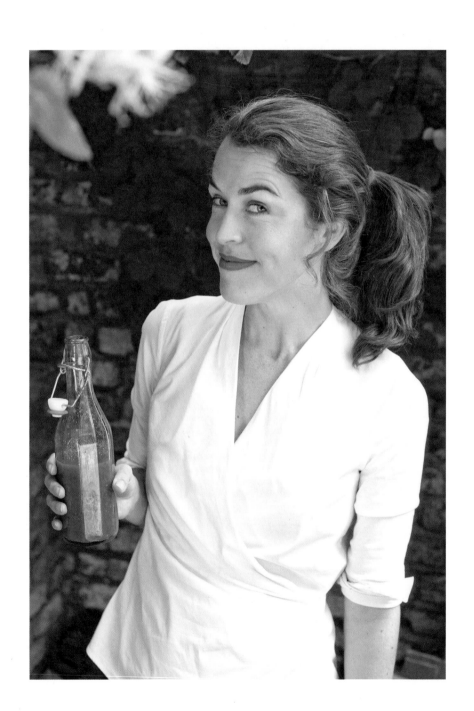

Introduction

FALLING DOWN THE RABBIT HOLE

My name is Susan Jane. Picture MacGyver in an apron with a grumpy
husband who thinks he's a restaurant critic and two ravenous little
punks to feed six times a day. Food is my thing, it keeps me happy.
People say my energy level would rival Serena Williams on acid.
But I wasn't always so bionic.

Thirteen years ago I was a college student in Dublin, and later at
Oxford University. Juggling deadlines, booze-ups, and tutorials was
a skill in itself. If I could fit them all in without expiring, surely
I was doing fine, right?

Looking back, I could never get enough sugar hits; I was an addict.
Everything I did related to or led to my next sugar fix. I even
convinced myself that college projects required gallons of coffee and
pounds of Curly Wurlies to charge my brain cells, that I couldn't
possibly perform without them.

Sound familiar?

I never saw myself as someone who needed to change. After all, there
was nothing out of the ordinary about my "Western" diet: jam-filled
scones, toast, pasta, breakfast cereals, toast, take-out
sandwiches, and more toast. Standard Irish fare. No wonder I tried
to regulate my moods with criminal amounts of caffeine.

Let's be honest: consumers are highly submissive. I hardly thought to ask any questions about the ingredients in my energy drink or the Monster Munch I devoured with the giddy determination of a meter maid spotting a Bentley in the bus lane. I blindly trusted the "food authorities," whoever they were, and I never imagined that beef burgers, for example, might contain horsemeat, that chicken products could test positive for pork, or that our modern diet would lead millions into "diabesity." Like Alice in Wonderland, I was jumping feet first into a deep, dark rabbit hole. Except this was no tea party.

First we form habits—and then they form us. It wasn't alcohol or cigarettes that ruined my health. It was food. Junk food. I convinced myself that only boring people had time to cook. Turns out, smarter people make time to cook.

One day in the summer of 2005 my body said no, enough. First came the shakes. Horrid urinary infections. Constipation. Mouth ulcers. Exhaustion. But nobody suggested that maybe I was contributing to my ill health. My digestive system wheezed like an asthmatic snail, yet diet apparently had nothing to do with it. Ten years ago the medical community dismissed the idea of food sensitivities like tycoons scoffing at global warming. Contemplating such an idea was daft. After all, test results had shown I was not celiac or diabetic. Case closed.

The chronic conditions started to make themselves at home. Thrush. Earaches. Dizziness. Psoriasis. Headaches. Cold sores. But I didn't have time to respect the symptoms and turned to self-medication. I had papers to submit. There was literally no time to be sick.

I ended up in the hospital, with tubes coming out of. . . well, every-where. They sent in doctor after doctor. As the consultants handed me their cards, I noticed the letters after their names kept getting longer and longer. Yet no one could figure out why my body was as limp as wet lettuce. I was numb, physically and emotionally.

After twelve courses of antibiotics, several hospitalizations, a course of steroids, anti-fungal colon treatments, and many futile vaccinations, I felt unlucky but in no way responsible. Then my white blood cells packed up.

One afternoon in the hospital, I got to chatting with an elderly lady called Lucy in the cubicle next to me. I wasn't certain why Lucy had been admitted. She was frail but so sweet in her papery mint gown, smiling back over the sheets. We talked for hours. I cried inside when she asked to hold my hand to give her strength. Lucy cooed about

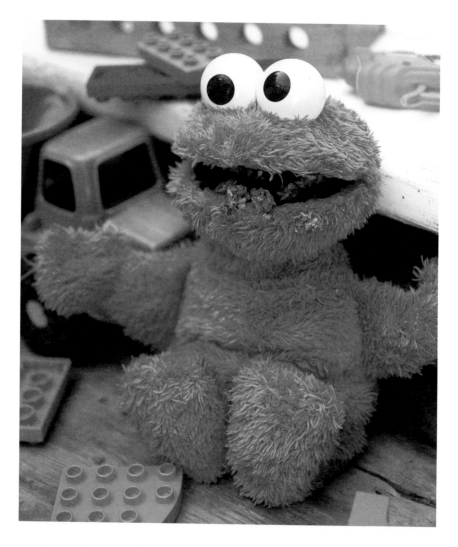

her love of bread making, yet she was celiac (so her body could not handle gluten). I remember thinking how strange that was: ignoring the signals her system was sending.

Across the room, another patient was tucking into jelly and ice cream from the hospital canteen. She was being treated for "complications" arising from diabetes and obesity. It was like death on a plate, and in a horribly ironic twist, the hospital staff were her accomplices. The sight sent a chill up my arms. Both women knew their poison but chose to ignore it. They were digging their way to their graves with their teeth. A little later, I heard a loud, flat bell. Doctors and nurses ran in and sectioned me off from Lucy. I never saw her adorable face again. No one did.

The following morning I looked in the mirror, and what I saw made me cry. I turned away from the mirror, and in that instant—a wrenching minute of pure self-knowledge, accompanied by a sort of grief for the person I was now saying good-bye to—I made the most important decision of my life: to take control of my health. Raising my head, I looked into that mirror once again. And I nodded.

Deal.

My nutritional pilgrimage started with a journey to Dr. Joe Fitzgibbon, an Irish GP who specializes in diet and fatigue. I traveled six hours by train for every visit. Together we tackled the Elimination Diet, stripping my meals to very basic foods like meat, fish, pulses, beans, and vegetables. It's not rocket science. In fact, it's pretty bloody obvious, right? But there's "nothing common about common sense," Dr. Fitzgibbon observed. Every couple of weeks I reintroduced specific foods to my diet to monitor symptoms, like a food detective. **It felt like someone was sucking the illness out of my body.**

That austere diet made me see the intimate connection between energy levels and the food we eat. Good food keeps you on your tippy toes. Poor food will have you on your knees. So I waved good-bye to all manner of processed food. That was ten years ago.

The first three weeks were horrific. I don't want you thinking I was running barefoot through fields of cornflowers, throwing my arms around trees in a state of orgasmic self-enlightenment. Nor did I ever choose to give up junk food. I had to. My body was falling apart. There was no other choice.

So I tramped around health food stores with a mixture of confusion and nervous elation, like an ornithologist sighting a new species of bird. All the time I was busy mourning for Diet Cola Girl. "Jesus, I could buy a bottle of wine for the price of that kombucha" and "I can't afford that weirdo flour, it's three times the price of the regular stuff!"

Eventually I realized there is nothing restrictive about this way of eating. It's the opposite. This was an empowering opportunity to escape the shackles of processed food and the excesses of the Wheat-Sugar-Dairy merry-go-round. **There are legions of grains, flours, and beans to experiment with in place of boring pasta and bread.** And instead of lobbing butter into my mouth ten times a day, I now discovered variety from a suite of other healthy fats like walnut, coconut, sesame, and hemp seed oils. Discovering this wealth of options was my second lightbulb moment. My "restrictive" diet was nothing of the sort. It was incredibly liberating.

By continuing to feed our bodies with one-dimensional foods made from white sugar, white flour, and industrially produced chemicals, we condition our brains to accept crap. Breaking the habit is challenging, but once you experience the benefit of eating whole, unprocessed foods, you will never look back. Make no mistake: it's a love affair like no other. But don't just take my word for it. See for yourself.

Eating well is intuitive. You already have the secret to wellness. You don't need a crew of neurotic food fascists on Instagram telling you what to eat. There are thousands of dynamite wholefoods to choose from. Herewith are my favorite recipes. Don't worry—I won't threaten you with cabbage soup or Lycra tights. These recipes are less about denial and more about pleasure: they are for joy-inducing foods, like banana malt ice cream, raw chocolate tortes, chestnut crêpes, smoky black bean bowls, spicy pomegranate noodles, and homemade pine nut ricotta. If you approach this book with a sense of adventure, I bet your palate will be tickled and your mojo will return. In time your weight will stabilize, you will sleep more soundly, and hum louder. But there's more! We now know that a healthy diet significantly reduces your risk of developing heart disease, many cancers, and type 2 diabetes. If there was a pill promising the same, wouldn't you want to take it? Whole-food cooking isn't a pill. It's a ticket.

Of course you shouldn't have to give up wheat, sugar, dairy, or any other food group in order to eat well. **Everyone has different needs and different poisons. That's what makes humans so damn charming.** For me, it's about expanding my choices—choices that I was never exposed to before. But whatever your reasons for exploring new and nourishing foods away from the circus of convenience, you are very welcome to my kitchen.

Let's do this together.

NIFTY Q&As

Do I need any special equipment before I start?

Definitely—get yourself some tenacity and a sense of adventure. Fleetwood Mac's *Greatest Hits* is also useful. Or Billie Holiday. Whatever tickles your serotonin.

Where do I buy all these weird things?

In good health food stores and specialist grocers. Most large supermarkets stock 80 percent of the ingredients listed, such as millet, quinoa, seaweed, tamari, and even coconut water. Check out my sources at the back of the book for online ordering.

How come you use cups instead of grams?

Cups are friendlier and make it easier to visualize quantities. I think the metric system alienates people in the kitchen. It has a disempowering effect. Do you know what 65 grams of dates looks like?

Or 325 grams of flour? You can pick up measuring cups in the baking aisle of most supermarkets or on Amazon. Dean & DeLuca probably does frilly ones. British and American cups differ, but don't panic—the difference is only 13 milliliters.

Why don't you use gluten-free flour?

I struggle to see the point of swapping white flour for a "gluten-free" version. It reminds me of when I used to drink decaf coffee, thinking I was being healthy. Gluten-free white flour is just as processed as its first cousin, the all-purpose white flour.

Admittedly, whole-grain flours are a little trickier to tame into happy cookies and breads, but their nutritional profile makes them much more desirable. If you've met my husband, you'll understand why I'm attracted to stubborn and contrary ingredients.

I find them indecently exciting once you finally conquer them.

Are all your recipes gluten-free as well as wheat-free?

Not all, but most. Gluten is found in wheat, rye, barley, and some oats.

Why don't you use spelt?

Spelt is wheat. Don't get me wrong—I eat spelt *and* wheat. But the idea of this cookbook is to introduce you to new foods.

If this cookbook is wheat-free, why does it feature lots of buckwheat recipes?

Despite its name, buckwheat is no relation to the cereal wheat. There's no gluten in buckwheat either. How awesome is that?

Any pasta recipes?

No. But plenty of quinoa, which is far tastier. It's like a new friend with superhuman powers. Pasta would blush in quinoa's presence.

Ground almonds are the same as almond flour, right?

Almost. Both are healthy and come from almonds, but ground almonds give a heavier finish in baked goodies. Almond flour is much finer and easier to find in the United States, but not so much in Europe.

Feel free to try almond flour in place of ground almonds whenever you see a recipe bound for the oven. However, almond flour will not work so well in any raw recipe, such as the Chia Bonbons, Hazelnut and Raisin Freezer Cookies, or Fancy Pants Lúcuma Fudge.

Is margarine OK instead of butter?

Not in my opinion. Be skeptical of pseudo foods tailored to "reduce cholesterol." Investigative journalist Felicity Lawrence warns that many manufacturers use the cheapest possible oils to make margarine and

hide under the pretense of being "healthy." Most of these oils must be processed or hydrogenated to extend their shelf life, but not your life. "Cholesterol-free" is a similarly deceptive marketing device among companies that use hydrogenated fats. So an ostensibly healthy product can do more harm to your cholesterol than good. Dr. Walter Willett, a professor at Harvard Medical School, slammed this as "the biggest food-processing disaster in US history."

How about regular sunflower oil?

For taste reasons, you're welcome to use whatever oil you fancy. However, as a cautious mummy of two growing boys I use only extra virgin, cold-pressed oils that have not been brutalized by processors or adulterated by manufacturers. When in doubt, leave it out.

Isn't coconut oil fattening?

It is a fat, yes. But it's a good fat. Our relationship with fat is perverse. We need it in order to manufacture brain cells and hormones (without which everyone

would be suffering from depression). However, choose judiciously. There are good fats and bad fats. Extra virgin, cold-pressed coconut oil is a good fat.

The saturated fat in coconut is made up of medium-chain triglycerides (MCTs), the mere mention of which makes triathletes indecently excitable. These MCTs are metabolised quickly by the body and can be used as an alternative source of energy to carbohydrates. MCTs are also easier to break down than the longer-chain triglycerides in olive, sunflower, and canola oils. More importantly, coconut's MCTs are composed of lauric and capric acids. These heroic antiviral, antifungal and antibacterial agents are also present in mother's milk to give her baba the best start in life.

Can I fry with olive oil?

Frying at a high temperature will denature almost any oil. It doesn't matter if you use the best cold-pressed extra virgin oil money can buy. Heating, as opposed to warming, chemically disfigures oil and spoils many health

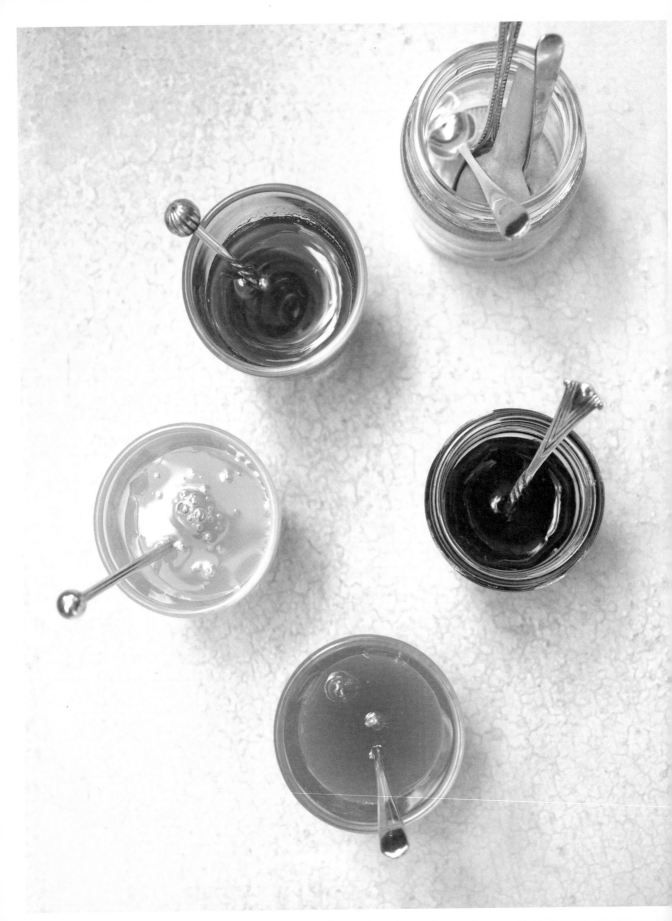

benefits. Basically, you are creating unhealthy free radicals that are liable to fraternize with your arteries. If you suffer from cholesterol or weight problems, it might be worth writing this on the inside of your kitchen cupboard to remind you!

We use coconut oil because of its high smoke point. This means it's a sturdier oil to cook with than, say, flaxseed or sunflower oil. When I'm gently sweating veggies, I'm happy to use olive oil, as the heat never reaches a perilous point.

Ghee is clarified butter, which many lactose-intol- erant cooks find they can eat without side effects. Just like butter, ghee is solid at room temperature and holds a higher smoke point than most oils. We always have some in our fridge.

I love agave and use
it all the time.
Is it good for me?

Let's be clear—no sugar is healthy. Agave is touted as a low-glycemic fructose syrup that does not require insulin to break it down. A health boon, right? But science is rarely that simple. Eating this page wouldn't

require insulin either. Hardly a reason to include it in our diet. It's fair to say that agave is not a health food but a useful food. This is an important differentiation. Evidence suggests that a diet rich in liquid fructose has a deleterious effect on the body. The addition of high-fructose corn syrup (HFCS), for example, has caused much controversy between health scientists and food manufacturers. While agave does not fall within the same category as HFCS, it is still classified as fructose.

Agave wouldn't be my first choice of sweetener unless I was diabetic (and even still, moderation is critical). Issues to consider include processing methods and added ingredients. Agave piracy dates back to 2008, when several supermarket brands of agave were found to be highly processed and contaminated with other forms of syrups. It's hardly surprising that manufacturers want a slice of success when a new food enjoys such attention. This applies to all newfangled foods. Keep your antennae finely tuned and your gut on speaking terms with you! As with all sweeteners,

no matter what you choose, moderation is key.

What's so terrific about
maple syrup anyway?
Isn't it just as bad
for you as sugar?

No. Unless you plan to neck a pint of it. Maple syrup is a wonderfully wholesome natural sugar. But if you're diabetic, it's off limits.

Maple syrup is harvested naturally from maple trees and contains surprising amounts of iron and calcium. It's one of the only sweeteners that helps alkalize the body—other sugars can be highly acidic to the system. Acidic systems have been shown to leach calcium from our bones, while alkaline systems actually enhance calcium absorption. This is useful information for those who suffer from arthritic or osteo conditions.

A pal in *Québec* is struggling to find local maple syrup. Rumor has it the middle-class Chinese are buying up all of Canada's stocks. This has consequences for us too, one of which is a rise in the price of this deliciously sticky nectar. Another is the surge of imposters on the market. To avoid being duped by "maple-flavored" syrup, always interrogate the labeling. It should have one ingredient: 100% pure Canadian maple syrup. Grade B is preferable.

What's the story with brown rice syrup? Healthy or not?

OK, so, no sugar is healthy. The key is to find one that works for you and use it moderately or sparingly.

Despite brown rice syrup being a fairly processed product, it has low levels of glucose (about 5%) and high levels of the more complex carbohydrate maltose (around 55%). This gives brown rice syrup an attractive glycemic load. Alicia Silverstone, author of The Kind Diet, totally digs it. As a result, Hollywood does too.

It's made by fermenting the cooked grain with cultured enzymes to break down the carbohydrates. The liquid by-product is boiled to make a sweet, sticky syrup. Like all trendy products, there are good versions and seriously processed versions. It's worth doing your own research. Sticking to organic seems

sensible given the volume of agrichemicals used in rice production. There were issues with arsenic in the soil a few years back too.

What on earth is coconut sugar?

Coconut blossom sugar is a relatively new unrefined sugar on the Western market. Stunning stuff. Not as sweet as regular cane sugar, it offers a burnt toffee kick. It's not heavily processed either. The sap of the coconut flower is dehydrated to form honeyed crystals. While coconut sugar can be classified as a palm sugar, it is not to be confused with regular palm sugar, which is produced differently and is no friend to the diabetic. Coconut sugar is thought to have a low glycemic value. Good news for hyperactive children, diabetics, and bored sedentary workers.

But watch out! My cynical side predicts that adulterated forms will begin to appear on our shelves. Look for trusted brands and ask your local health food stockist for advice if you're suspicious. Coconut sugar is pricey and will attract piracy. Them is the facts of life. Rapadura sugar

is much more difficult to adulterate and is a very good sub for coconut sugar if glycemic load does not concern you.

If rapadura is cane sugar, what's it doing in this book?

You'll notice that rapadura sugar features in just three recipes. I wanted to introduce readers to a range of healthier sugars in place of the nutritionally void white variety.

Rapadura is a unique extra-fine sugar made from dehydrating sugarcane juice. It is caramel in color with a deep mineral taste to it. Find it online and in all good food stores. Pricey, but worth experiencing.

However, if your diet obliges you to stay off sugar, this would mean quarantining all forms of good and bad sugars, including rapadura, honey, maple syrup, brown rice syrup, and even fruit. My cookbook only manages to evict nasty white sugar from our kitchens.

I'm diabetic.
Is this book for me?

Absolutely. However, it's important to stick to your low GL principles. Wherever you see maple syrup, use raw agave or experiment with xylitol. Coconut sugar is apparently low GL, but at the time of going to print, there was insufficient independent research to corroborate this for me. I urge you to do your own research. Remember that dried fruit, date syrup, maple syrup, apple syrup, and honey are all high on the glycemic index and therefore unsuitable. Stevia is an interesting and popular source of sweetness for many diabetics, but I don't like the taste. Perhaps you will have better luck than me.

Can I use barley malt extract in place of maple syrup? It's so much cheaper.

Sure. Although I haven't tried barley malt in all my recipes, I can assure you it gives tremendous results in baking. Even raw chocolates work with barley malt. Just remember that it's only half as sweet as honey and maple syrup. This syrup is made from fermenting and boiling barley, in a similar way to brown rice syrup. Some of the original nutrients found in barley are transferred to the nectar. While barley malt is not as sweet as maple syrup, it's unusually malty and licky-sticky.

Barley malt is a complex sugar, meaning that it takes quite some time for it to be broken down by the body. Simple sugars, like white sugar or corn syrup, are absorbed immediately, resulting in blood sugar spikes and yo-yo moods. For evidence of this, spend thirty minutes at a children's birthday party. It's pretty mental.

Cutting out convenience food is difficult. How can I cope with cooking all the time?

With great music, the sort that makes your blood pelt around your body and electrifies your fingertips. Nothing is a chore when your favorite tunes massage your neurotransmitters. It's key to cooking. I also throw lots of suppers and treats into my freezer, ready to plunder on lazy days. Be selfish with your time—conquer many meals in one session, rather than cooking three times a day. With practice, you'll motor through these recipes.

How do I know if I have a food intolerance?

If you've already bought this book, chances are something's not agreeing with you. Find a registered dietician or doctor to do an elimination diet with you. I'm not a huge fan of allergy testing, simply because it didn't bring any relief to me. For best results, become your own food detective (with the encouragement of and direction from a professional).

Why are soy and tofu controversial? I'm confused. Are they the same thing?

Tofu is made from soy beans. You're probably familiar with other soy bean products, such as soy milk, miso soup, soy sauce, and tempeh. Milk is extracted from the soy bean and used to make soy curd, referred to as tofu. It's not unlike cheese making. Made this way, tofu is supposedly replete with isoflavones, a big pal of calcium. Isoflavones have been found to assist in bone density as well as hormonal imbalances. So far, so good.

Once soy's health benefits became clear outside of Japan, consumer demand rocketed. I think its explosive rise here in the West encouraged food companies to find cheaper ways of producing it. Consequently, soy's reputation has been muddied with chemical isolation techniques, synthetic adulteration, and genetic modification, all of which raise serious questions about the beneficial effects of the end product. That's why soy is so controversial. The chemically altered soy is a whole different creature to the whole-bean soy associated with the Asian diet. Frustrating, isn't it?

The only way you can tell the difference is to read the manufacturer's label on food before you buy. I've been advised to avoid soy protein isolates. Up to 60 percent of packaged supermarket foods use this synthetically debased soy as a cheap bulking agent. So don't be fooled into thinking soy is synonymous with health.

To tap into soy beans' bona fide health benefits, my advice is to stick with organic, non-GM tofu and eat it no more than once a week. Even the Japanese don't eat as much soy as we do. There are also ethical issues to consider. Animal feed is composed largely of soy, which drives demand for soy plantations. We are witnessing the destruction of hundreds of thousands of wildlife acres to satiate demand for soy production. In short, the world has gone bonkers for the stuff. If you can live without it, all the better.

Do you eat Quorn?

Nope, never. Cutting down on meat seems to be a much more sensible approach. Swapping one bad habit for another makes little sense.

Are these recipes suitable for children?

Definitely. Just leave out the salt, black pepper, garlic, or tamari—and add these to your own plate. Good nutrition is the best health insurance you can offer your family.

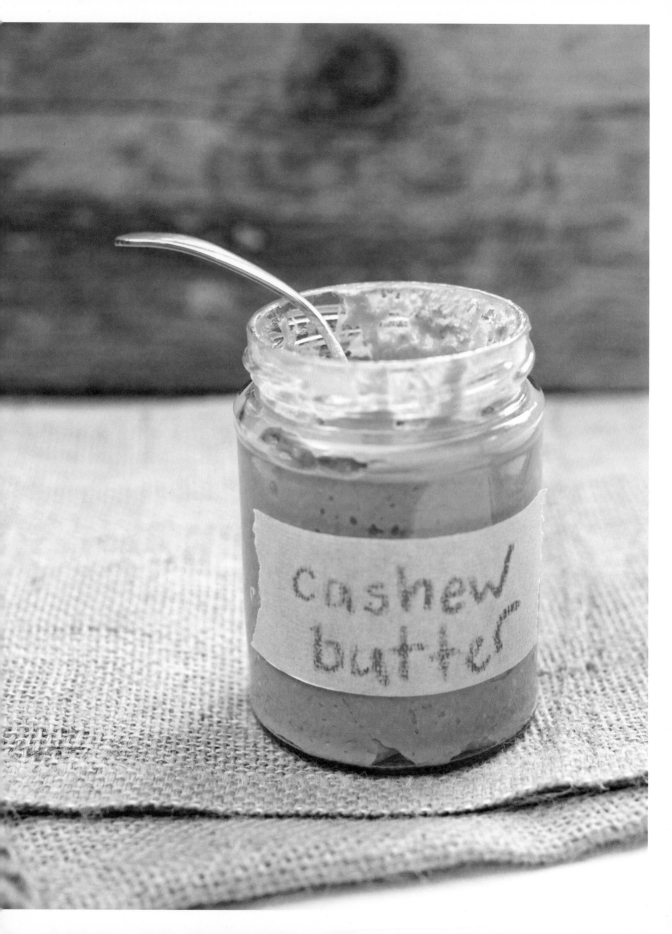

YOUR KITCHEN'S ARTILLERY

****

HERE ARE YOUR NEW ALLIES IN THE KITCHEN, IN ORDER OF IMPORTANCE.

Measuring cups

You'll notice I measure in cups, handfuls, and drizzles, which makes it easier to visualize quantities as you read the recipe and write your shopping list. I've always found grams and ounces alienating. It may as well be trigonometry to me. Like most tactile people, I function on a sort of visual mathematics. We use British/Australian cups where 1 cup = 250 milliliters. American cups measure 237 milliliters, only a touch smaller.

Pestle and mortar

If you don't have a pestle and mortar, find an Asian food store. You'll pick up an excellent deal, save yourself a small fortune, and instantly acquire bragging rights at the bar. A pestle and mortar propels you into an underground club of serious cooks. Think Jamie Oliver meets Thomas Keller. No good meal can be made without a bit of muscle action in the kitchen. I guess the bottom of a heavy saucepan would also work, but it might scare the bejesus out of the neighbors.

Food processor

Mine's a Magimix from my mother-in-law. The lady's got style. I use it every day.

Hand-held or personal blender

Also referred to as a soup gun or whizzy thing, hand-held blenders give a much smoother finish than a food processor (unless you have a swanky Vitamix). Particularly important for hummus (page 114). Pick one up for around 25 bucks.

Heavy-based saucepan or large sauté pan

Heavy-based saucepans spread heat evenly, which helps prevent burning or ingredients "catching" on the bottom of the pan and driving your patience batty. Le Creuset are the Bentleys of the kitchen. Look out for them during sale season or in discount stores like T.J. Maxx. The bigger, the better.

Oven thermometer

This is like a lie detector for ovens. Available online on Amazon and in kitchen stores.

Spiralizer

Mine is a Lurch, and it's definitely love. Not essential to your kitchen, it's more of a nerdy toy.

Tefal 8-in-1 Multi Cooker

To make perfectly fluffy quinoa, measure 2 cups of quinoa to level 2 in the basin. Season with a few turns of the sea salt and peppercorn mill. Press the "grains" setting. The cooker will steam the grain and produce the most perfect quinoa you're ever likely to taste.

For details on how to cook almost every brown rice on the market using this cooker, visit my blog at www.susanjanewhite.com.

Empty jam jars

To transport food into work with you and be the envy of all your coworkers.

Tenacity

Available deep down, often in the same aisle as drive and desperation.

Ideas for Breakfast

"Keep your face to the sunshine,
and you will never see the shadows."
—Helen Keller

The breakfast roll is dead. Who wants to hoover up chemically
enhanced meat, bleached rolls, and puddles of cholesterol?

We've designed this chapter for anyone who dreads the
shrill of their alarm clock. Some recipes involve a little forward
planning but will ultimately gift you with more snoozage and
go-go juice (the High-Octane Banana Nutmeg Bars
on page 34 last all week in the fridge, for example).

Only six seconds to fuel up? No problem. Stick your hand in the
freezer to loot your store of ready-made goodies from this book:
Lemon and Pistachio Pie (page 224), Office Bombs (page 62),
Your New Wheat-Free Bread (page 51), Goji Berry Halva (page 207),
Strawberry Shortbread (page 231), Blackberry Tart (page 235),
Flaxseed Focaccia (page 54), Barley Grass Balls (page 66),
or Chia Bonbons (page 64).

I swear you won't miss your breakfast cereal and milk.
In fact, I bet you'll look back on your favorite cereal packet like
a bad ex and wonder what on earth you ever saw in it.
It was a love affair controlled by a sugar rush, and little else.
Good riddance.

**Visit page 12 to learn more about my alternatives to
refined cane sugar.**

THE ONLY GRANOLA RECIPE YOU'LL EVER NEED

****

A bowl of DIY granola and nut milk is a great way to start the day. It takes just twenty minutes to make, and the benefits last all week. The beauty of making your own granola is the satisfaction of knowing exactly what went into it-none of the cheap fats, preservatives, sugar, or gunk regularly found in commercial ones.

For your inner Mary Poppins, tie a ribbon around a jar of granola, and surprise someone.

2 cups nuts (260 g) nuts (pecans, walnuts, Brazil nuts, hazelnuts)

2¹/₂ cups (225 g) jumbo oats

1 cup (100 g) quinoa flakes

1 cup (130 g) combination of sunflower and pumpkin seeds

5 tablespoons ground flaxseeds or ground almonds

1 teaspoon sea salt flakes

³/₄ cup (190 ml) raw honey or maple syrup

³/₄ cup (190 ml) extra virgin coconut oil

Grated zest of 1 orange

2 cups (280 g) dried fruit (cranberries, dates, raisins, unsulfured apricots)

1 rough cup (100 g) dried banana, chopped

Makes 20 servings

Preheat the oven to 340°F (170°C). Line 2 baking trays with parchment paper.

Roughly chop any big nuts (pecans are fine left whole). Toss the nuts in a large bowl with the oats, quinoa flakes, seeds, ground flaxseeds and salt. Feeling adventurous? A tablespoon of cinnamon or dried ginger will add another flavor layer.

Gently warm the honey, oil, and orange zest together. Pour over the bowl of oats and coat well. You won't be adding the dried fruit until after baking.

Spread thinly on the baking trays and transfer to the middle shelf of the oven. Bake for 17-20 minutes. Shake the trays after 8 minutes to prevent burning. You're aiming for a light golden color. Oats and nuts taste bitter if you let them turn brown.

Remove from the oven and allow to cool and solidify completely before tossing through the dried fruit. Store in an airtight container for 2-3 weeks. Great with the Brazil nut milk on page 75 or cultured coconut yogurt. Makes enough to last all week for a large family.

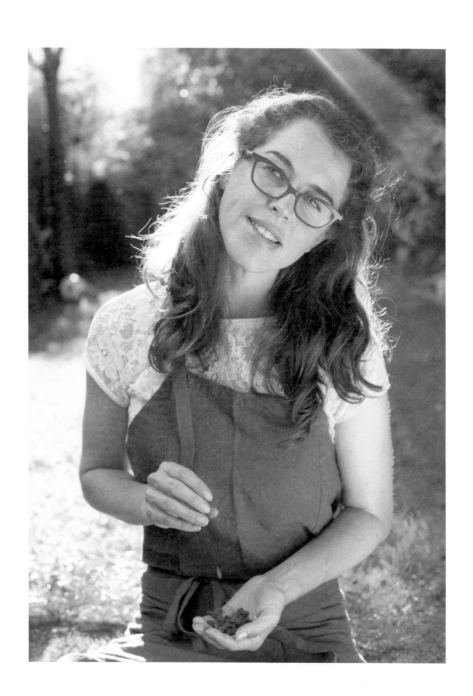

MANGO, BLACKBERRY, AND BUCKWHEAT PORRIDGE

****

This is no ordinary porridge. But then again, this is no ordinary cookbook. Every recipe is designed to feed your battery and have you high-jumping those afternoon slumps.

Despite its name, buckwheat is not related to wheat and does not contain gluten. That's a high-five and a backflip for celiacs.

¹/₂ cup (100 g) buckwheat
  grain, soaked overnight
Squeeze of lemon juice
1 small apple, grated
A bite-size chunk of coconut
  cream*
¹/₂ mango, sliced (or soak
  some dried mango overnight)
Handful of blackberries
  (optional)
Maple or apple syrup, to serve

Serves 1

You can use coconut milk in place of water, but it works out to be a lot more expensive. Coconut cream comes in a block, and you can chip off bits as you need it. Just store it in the fridge.

Soak the buckwheat overnight in water and a squeeze of lemon juice. In the morning, pour off the excess water (and debris), then rinse in a sieve to separate the grains once more. This process breaks down the phytic acid in the cereal and makes it more digestible as well as quicker to cook.

Bring 1 cup of water to a boil. Add the soaked buckwheat, grated apple, and the shavings or chunks of coconut cream. Cook for 15–20 minutes at a put-putter rather than a ferocious boil. It will thicken and become creamy with time.

Best adorned with juicy mango slivers, messy black-berries, and DIY apple syrup (see page 25). While mangos can be pricey, you can sniff out massive boxes of them in Asian stores every June, July, and August for buttons. Soaked dried mango works for the rest of the year.

METRO MUESLI WITH CHIA JAM

****

Rushed for breakfast? Time for muesli making, darling. Not that fancy expensive stuff you pass wistfully in trendy delis. I mean your very own creations, transported in a snazzy jar with a spoon, appetite, and sleepy smile. It will make your commute actually enjoyable.

Oats don't always have to be eaten as molten-hot porridge. Soaking oat flakes overnight in a liquid (water, milk, apple juice) makes them delectably sweet and more digestible. Prepping this breakfast is an easy habit to acquire, sparing those brain cells first thing in the morning. But don't take my word for it. Try it and see.

Gastroenterologists—the specialists who look after your pipes—recommend getting 25 to 35 grams of dietary fiber every day. A bowl of Metro Muesli with Chia Jam will give you an almighty 22 grams of fiber before the day even dawns. Add grated apple for an extra 5 grams or banana for 3 grams. Want to know the average daily intake in Ireland? A measly 10 grams. (It's 16 grams in the United States.) Highly processed diets are devoid of fiber. Given that colon cancer and heart disease are top killers, it's probably time to make friends with a new breakfast regime.

This is just a variation on Bircher muesli. Stir all the ingredients together except the cinnamon. Use whatever ingredients on hand that you feel really work for you—a tablespoon of buckwheat? Blueberries? Grated apple? Cacao nibs? Banana? Hazelnuts? The following morning, scoop into a jar and crown with cinnamon before you dash out the door. Don't forget a spoon.

If you have the time, try making some chia jam. It's a quirky variation on the sugar-laden stuff. Defrost the berries, and blend with the lemon and chia. Leave the mixture to soak for 20 minutes or overnight before spooning on top of your muesli. Store in a jam jar for up to 3 days. Ta-da!

For the muesli:
$^2/_3$ cup (60 g) jumbo oats
$^1/_3$ cup (50 g) raisins
1 cup (250 ml) water, apple
  juice, soy or nut milk
2 tablespoons flaxseeds
Squeeze of lemon juice
Sprinkle of pumpkin seeds
Sprinkle of sunflower seeds
Sprinkle of ground cinnamon

Serves 1

For the chia jam:
1 cup frozen cherries or
  blackberries, defrosted
Sqeeze of lemon juice
2 tablespoons chia seeds

Makes 6-8 servings

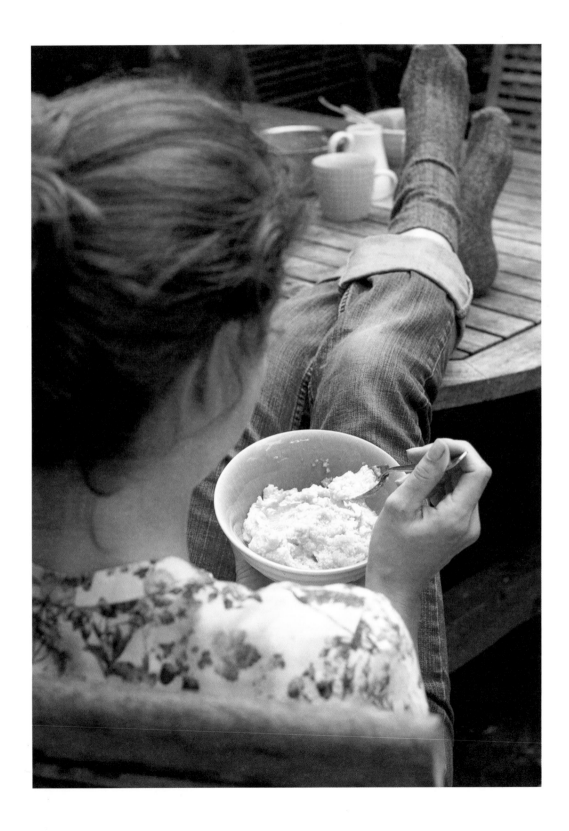

DECENT MILLET PORRIDGE AND APPLE SYRUP

****

Millet is not a fabulously tasty grain. My nostrils balked and my palate winced the first time I made porridge with it. But by teaming millet with strong flavors, you'll bring out this grain's best quality: its texture.

Millet's nutritional kudos and affordability are good enough reasons to introduce it to your breakfast table. Sprinkle with coconut blossom sugar for the food nerd in you, but living in Ireland means I'm able to get my hands on Highbank Orchard Syrup. This is our answer to maple syrup, made from 100 percent local organic apples and love.

Cook the millet and water over medium heat for 3-5 minutes before adding the creamed corn and salt. That's it!

To make your own apple syrup, boil the juice for 25 minutes until it resembles a viscous syrup. Store in an airtight jar and summon when required. Ideally, you'll need to use fresh apple syrup within 4-5 days.

This delicious sticky nectar is rich in potassium, the mineral that helps evacuate hangovers. Just saying.

For the porridge:
$1/3$ cup (40 g) millet flakes
$2/3$ cup (165 ml) water
$1/3$ cup (75 g) puréed sweetcorn
Pinch of salt flakes

Serves 1

For the apple syrup:
4-6 cups unsweetened or fresh
  apple juice

Makes 6-8 servings

DOUBLE DECKER AMARANTH AND BANANA PUD

****

Amaranth is another one of those supergrains that have the Hollywood glitterati genuflecting. It has serious nutritional gravitas, rivaling quinoa as the number one seed. Amaranth's got more muscle than wheat, clocking in four times the amount of calcium and twice as much iron. And with generous stores of lysine, you can kiss cold sores toodle-oo. Not bad for half a cent per gram.

A caveat for the cook: bananas used in this recipe need to be overripe. Any green areas on the banana skin means they have not ripened fully and will make the pudding bitter. Look for older bananas with blackened sweet spots.

Please don't try this recipe with coconut milk or almond milk. Something offensive happens.

1 cup (200 g) amaranth grain
1¹/₂ cup (375 ml) water
¹/₄ teaspoon sea salt
3 tablespoons maple syrup
3 tablespoons tahini or
  almond butter
2 large eggs, beaten
2 cups (500 ml) soy, hemp,
  or oat milk
2 very ripe bananas, chopped
¹/₂ cup (75 g) raisins
1 teaspoon vanilla extract
1 tablespoon rapadura or
  coconut sugar
1 tablespoon ground cinnamon

Serves 6-8

Preheat the oven to 325°F (160°C).

In a small saucepan with a tight-fitting lid, bring the amaranth, water, and salt to a soft boil. This means a gentle putter rather than a violent bubble that will blow the lid off and scare the bejesus out of your budgie. Cook for 15 minutes, until the water is fully absorbed. Amaranth is not a dry, fluffy grain when cooked. Expect something that looks like a gluey couscous.

While the amaranth is doing its thing, prep the rest of the gear. Blend the maple syrup and nut butter together until smooth, then add the eggs. Pour this mixture into the milk and add the chopped bananas, raisins, and vanilla.

Remove the amaranth from the heat, stir briskly and add in the milky mixture. Give it all a gentle stir.

Pour and scrape the pudding mix into a medium-size pie dish (about the size of a magazine page). You're aiming for a pudding at least 1 inch deep, but no more than 2 inches. Pyrex rectangular glass dishes give the best result for custardy puds like this one. Cook for 40 minutes in a conventional oven. It should wobble slightly in the center when removed. Halfway through cooking, mix together the rapadura sugar and cinnamon and sprinkle it on top.

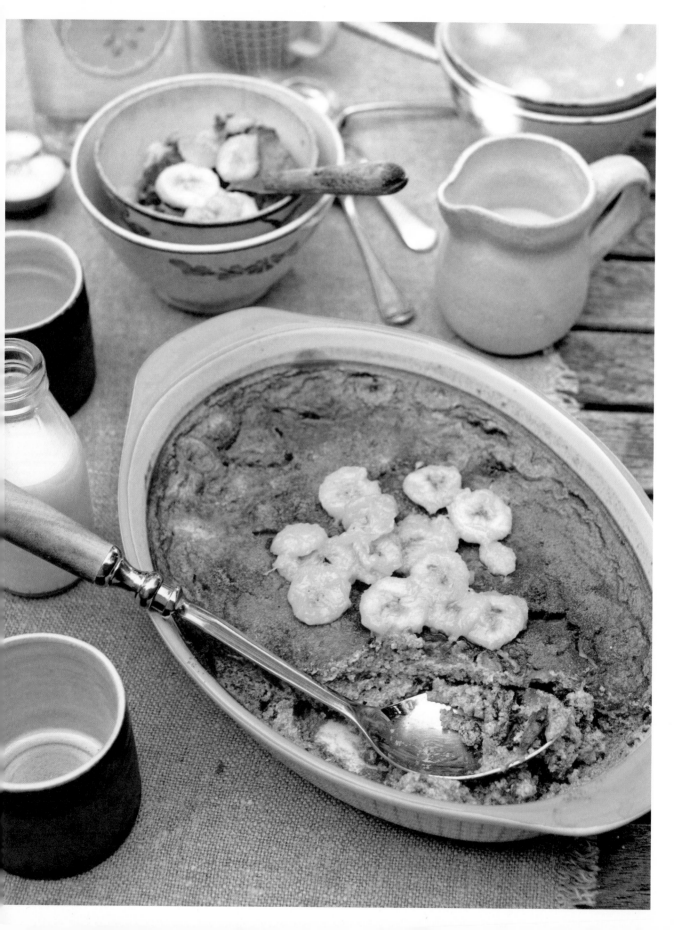

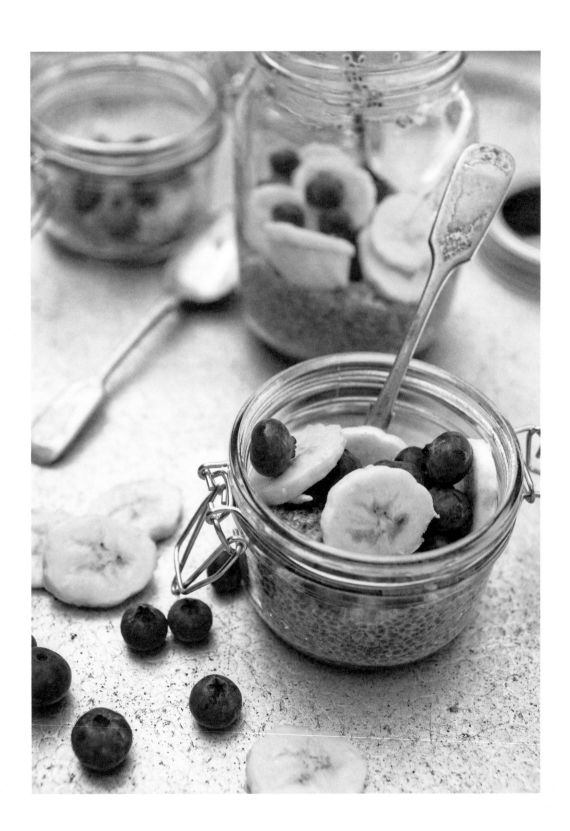

CHIA AND CHAI BREAKFAST PUDDING

****

I make this for my little monsters and their mighty appetites. While chai tea is not essential, I recommend using it through the wintry months. Sweet chai contains cardamom, cinnamon, ginger, anise, fennel, and cloves-all of which are warming spices for your belly.

Using a fork, whisk together the chia seeds, milk, and mashed banana. Tear open the sweet chai tea bag and stir it through. Allow the chia pudding to set overnight, either in the fridge or on the countertop. Serve in the morning with blueberries. A sneaky drizzle of brown rice syrup is awfully good too.

$^3/_4$ cup (125 g) chia seeds
2 cups (500 ml) almond
  (or other) milk
1 tea bag of sweet chai
  (or cinnamon)
1 banana, mashed
Handful of blueberries
Drizzle of brown rice syrup
  (optional)

Serves 4

BADASS BREAKFAST BARS

****

These fiber-rich breakfast bars are sure to have your arteries applauding. No butter, cream, sugar, or stodgy white flour—just pure, unadulterated whole foods the way Mother N intended. The attraction of low-glycemic food like oats is that it breaks down slowly, releasing a steady stream of energy into the body. Picture drip-feeding your diesel tank so that it never runs empty. This makes oats an excellent diabetic food, but also gold for athletes, weight watchers, hyper children, and anxious politicians.

More geek speak? Oats' cargo of soluble and insoluble fiber has the nifty ability to service our pipes in more ways than one. There ain't nothing sexy about consti-pation, especially given that our skin often takes over as an excretory organ. Yes, oats will make you regular, but they'll also escort cholesterol out of your body like a bad-tempered bodyguard.

It's important to note that oats need to be cooked or soaked in order to tap into their nutritional benefits. Muesli straight out of a bag with milk does not count.

4 ¹/₂ cup (670 g) combination of dried apricots, prunes and pitted dates

Juice of 1 lime

4 tablespoons pumpkin seeds (optional)

5 cups (450 g) oat flakes*

1 cup (100 g) ground almonds

1 cup (140 g) rye flour*

¹/₂ cup (50 g) ground chia or ground flaxseeds

1 teaspoon unrefined organic salt

1 cup (250 ml) freshly squeezed orange juice

1 cup (250 ml) extra virgin coconut oil

5 tablespoons barley malt extract, maple syrup, or brown rice syrup*

Makes 20-25 bars

* For the gluten-sensitive brigade, I find using brown rice flour, maple syrup, and gluten-free oats works well.

Preheat the oven to 350°F (180°C). Line an 8 x 8-inch baking pan (or something similar) with parchment paper.

Place your apricots, prunes, and dates in a saucepan and pour in enough water to come just below the level of the fruit. Bring to a boil, then lower the heat and simmer for 15-20 minutes with the lid on. If steam escapes, add a touch more water. Once cooked, stir through the lime juice and mix until the fruits are almost smooth. Set aside.

While the fruits are doing their thing, briefly pulse the pumpkin seeds in a blender or a coffee grinder. You can chop them up with a sharp knife if you prefer less washing up, or buy them pre-milled.

In a mixing bowl (and wearing a deliciously frilly apron), mix together the pumpkin seeds, oats, ground almonds, rye flour, chia/flaxseeds, and salt. If your oats are big, pulse them in a food processor first with the pumpkin seeds. Finer oat flakes give better results, but be careful not to pulse into an oatmeal or flour.

(continued)

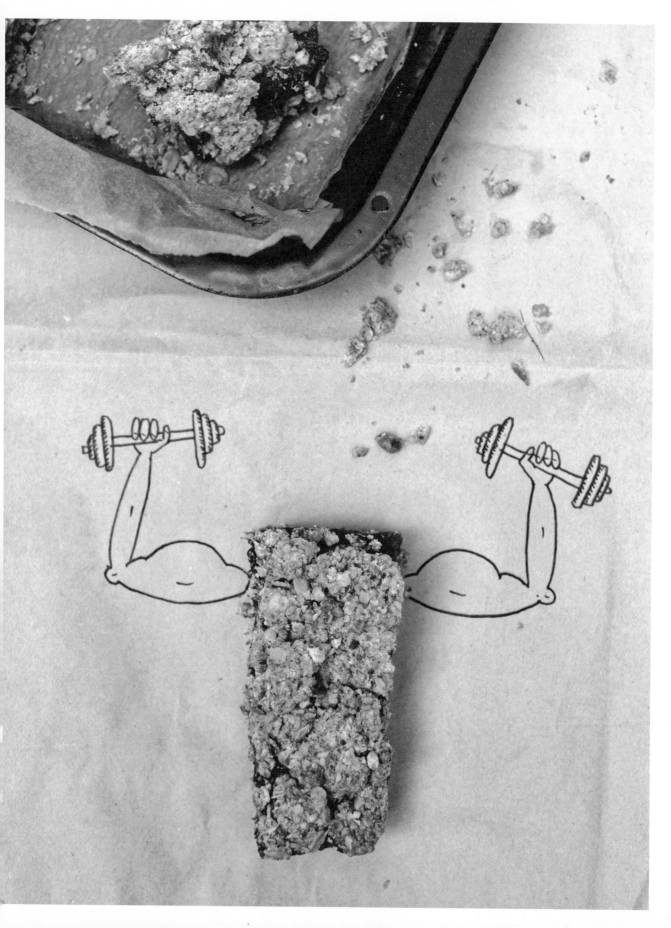

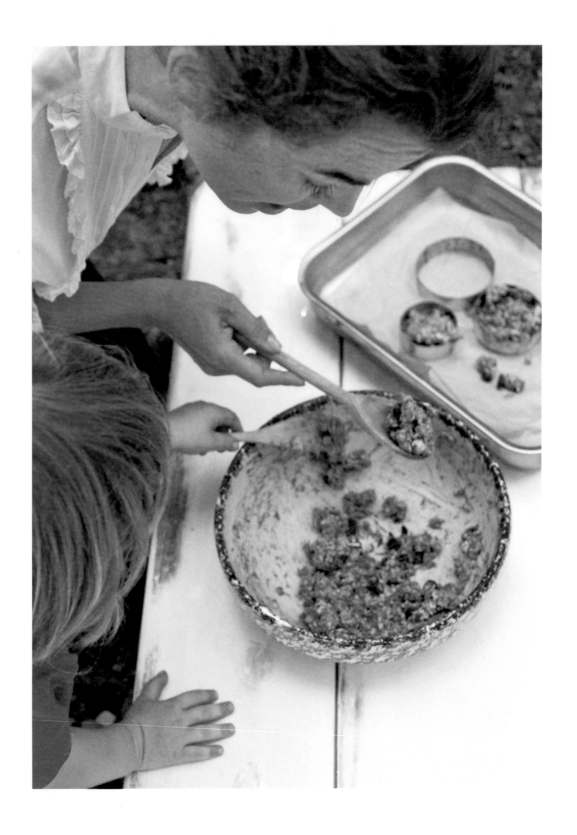

In a separate bowl, mix the orange juice, oil, and sweetener and pour into the dry ingredients, stirring until everything is glistening.

Using dampened fingers, press two-thirds of the oat mix into the lined pan. It's really gooey and sticky, so ramp up the radio to take the edge off impatient fingers. Spread the jammy apricot mix over this base. Gently press the remaining oat mix on top of the apricot mix. You'll need to do this with your fingers again. Take a curtsy-only if you're wearing a frilly apron, otherwise you'll look a bit silly-and admire your brilliance.

Place on the center shelf of the oven and bake for 40 minutes, until lightly golden but not browned. Allow to cool before slicing into squares. Store on top of paper towels inside an airtight tin or in the fridge. The smell of these Badass Breakfast Bars will draw children away from their Nintendo like the Pied Piper.

These keep well in the fridge for up to 10 days. In other words, a lot of happy breakfasts.

HIGH-OCTANE BANANA NUTMEG BARS

****

Commercial breakfast bars are full of sugar, cheap hydrogenated fat, and salt-none of which your brain cells will appreciate. With increasing financial pressure on producers to lower their production costs, it's hard to trust anything with a wrapper and a marketing department nowadays. These homemade breakfast bars are a healthy alternative and store really well in the fridge for 2 weeks.

Don't be put off by coconut oil's saturated fat content. These fats are in the form of medium-chain triglycerides. MCTs readily convert to energy, in contrast to longer-chain triglycerides such as sunflower oil. This is done through our cells' mitochondria-the gateway to our body's fuel. No wonder sports stars choose this oil over any other. What a shame no one told Lance Armstrong.

1 cup (150 g) Medjool dates or
  pre-soaked regular dates
2 cups (180 g) oats
1 cup (100 g) ground almonds
³/₄ cup (55 g) broken banana
  chips (not dried banana)
¹/₂ cup (65 g) chopped pecans
¹/₂ cup (75 g) raisins
Handful of sunflower seeds
1-2 teaspoons grated nutmeg
1 teaspoon sea salt flakes
³/₄ cup (190 ml) extra virgin
  coconut oil
¹/₂ cup (125 ml) honey,
  brown rice syrup, or barley
  malt extract

Makes 20 bars

Preheat the oven to 340°F (170°C). Line a pan no bigger than a magazine page with parchment paper.

Chop the dates and combine with the remaining dry ingredients in a large bowl. Merrily mix.

In a saucepan, gently melt the coconut oil with your choice of natural sweetener for around 5 minutes, until nicely melded. Strangely, maple syrup does not work in this recipe.

Create a hole in the center of your dry ingredients and add the deliciously syrupy coconut oil. Energetically mix, preferably with sashaying hips and a bit of Rolling Stones. This helps every last bit of your gooey mix to glisten. Pour into the prepared pan and press down firmly with your fingers. Licking of utensils and bowl most definitely encouraged. Lightens up the washing.

Bake for 35 minutes, until lightly golden-any darker in color and the oats will turn bitter. Remove from the oven and allow to rest for 10 minutes before refrigerating them. Resist cutting until they have chilled. Otherwise you will be left with a frustratingly messy affair, which no amount of Rolling Stones can remedy.

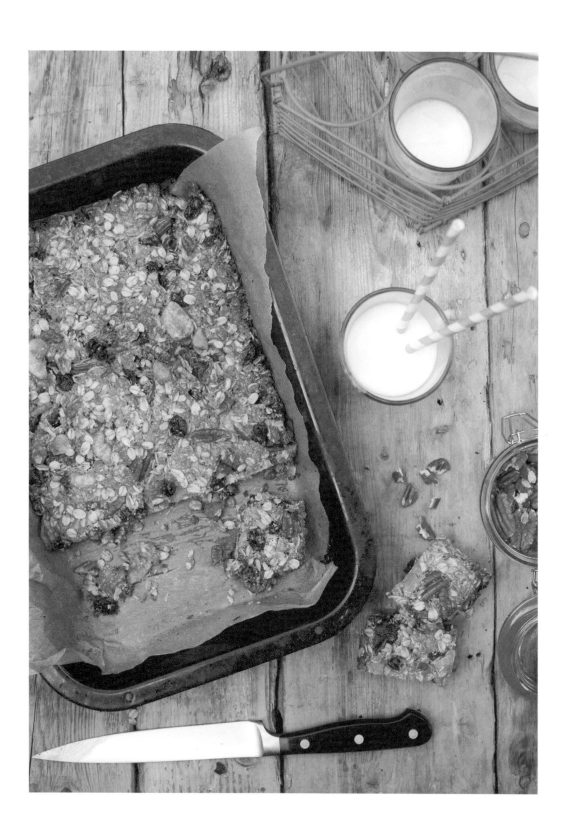

MAPLE AND CARDAMOM PEACHES

****

Peaches are bursting with vitamins that keep our bodies jolly. Niacin in particular helps improve circulation to the brain-something most of us would appreciate on a Sunday morning.

And you know the disappointing, fluffy peaches you sink your teeth into? Those infuriating peach imposters? No need to hurl them in the bin. Collect yourself, and scald the living daylights out of them instead. A peach's sweetness will sing once heated. Such delicious reprisal.

If you're using fresh ginger in place of dried ginger, try peeling a thumb-size piece and freezing until firm. This makes it super easy to grate and ensures the ginger's stringy fibers don't corrupt your brekkie. Grated frozen ginger gives any dish a heart-thumping ping-my number one tip for boring lentils and despondent salads.

4 massive peaches
2 tablespoons maple syrup
$1/_4$ teaspoon ground cardamom
$1/_2$ teaspoon fresh or dried
  ginger
Cultured soy or coconut
  yogurt, to serve
Squeeze of lemon juice,
  to serve

Serves 4-8

Preheat your grill or barbecue. It's wise to clean any residue from yesterday's messy chicken wings-not a good companion to today's breakfast.

Cut the peaches in half and remove the stone. This is noticeably easier with ripe peaches, as underripe peaches refuse to let loose their center stone. Then, using a lunchbox and lid, mix the maple syrup and spices together. Pop the peach halves inside and shake the box to coat the fruit.

Place the gooey, coated peaches on a grill or over the barbecue flames and cook for a few minutes on each side, depending on how hot it is. You'll be the judge of that. Remove each one gently, as they are decidedly delicate now. Dig in with yogurt and a spritz of lemon juice, or chill for up to 3 days in the fridge.

6 A.M. TODDLER COOKIES

****

Ever up at 6 a.m. with your teeny tots? These cookies will keep them quietly active while nourishing their little motors. There's hardly any mess-notice there's no flour or eggs.

Preheat the oven to 350°F (180°C). Line a baking tray with parchment paper.

Grate the apple into a large mixing bowl. If you're crafty enough to do this without getting your knuckles involved, high-five your toddler. Toss through the remaining ingredients, coating everything really well with the mashed banana. Make approximately 16 cookies by taking a tablespoon of the dough and flattening it between your hands, just like Play-Doh.

Place on the lined baking tray and bake for 12 minutes, or a little longer if the cookies are a bit bigger. No need to cool on a wire rack-let them find your breakfast table immediately. Minor caveat-scarf them down all on the same day, as they tend to misbehave after 24 hours.

1 medium apple
1 cup (90 g) porridge oats
  (not jumbo)
$^1/_2$ cup (75 g) sultanas or
  raisins
$^1/_2$ cup (125 g) mashed banana
2 teaspoons baking powder
$^1/_2$ teaspoon ground cinnamon

Makes 16 cookies

STICKY CINNAMON AND PRUNE CAKES

****

Unless you were born before 1945, a prune cupcake sounds as appealing as a jug of turnip juice. But balk not. My friend the prune has more antioxidants than a blueberry. Prunes are a lot cheaper too. Add to this the nutritional superpowers of psyllium husks, apples, bananas, pecans, olive oil, carrots, cinnamon, and rye, and you've got yourself a love bomb. Just what your body needs to survive a morning in the office.

8 squishy prunes, destoned
  and chopped
1 medium banana, mashed
¹/₄ cup (30 g) pecans
Just under 1 cup (200 ml)
  unsweetened or fresh
  apple juice
4 tablespoons raw agave,
  maple or yacón syrup, or
  barley malt extract
2 tablespoons psyllium husks
4 tablespoons extra virgin
  olive oil
1 cup (60 g) loosely packed
  grated carrots
1¹/₄ cup (175 g) rye flour
2 teaspoons baking powder
1 teaspoon ground cinnamon

Makes 9 muffins

Preheat the oven to 350°F (180°C). Line a muffin tray with 9-12 paper cases.

In a large bowl, mix together the prunes, banana, pecans, apple juice, sweetener, flaxseeds, and oil. Stir through the grated carrots and set aside.

In a separate bowl, introduce the rye flour to the baking powder and cinnamon. Make sure the baking powder doesn't stick in one place. Make a well in the center of the flour and scoop the wet prune mixture into it. Mix thoroughly. I always find singing loudly helps. Spoon into your prepared muffin tray, but don't fill the cases too high or they won't cook in the center.

Bake for 30-35 minutes (or half that time if using a mini muffin tray). Remove from the oven and watch hungry nostrils dance. These muffins benefit from cooling down for 20 minutes to solidify and rest. Very difficult to resist looting, so remove self from kitchen and find distraction elsewhere.

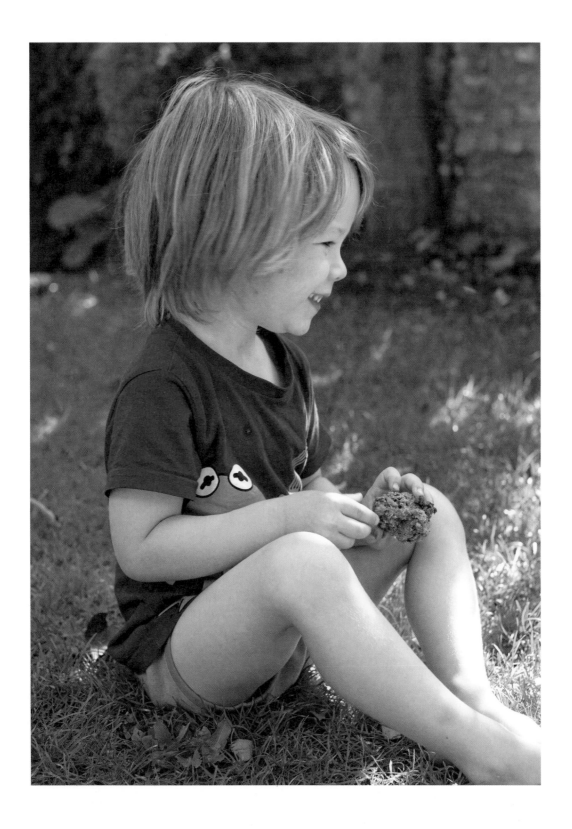

SCRAMBLED TOFU WITH CARAMELIZED ONION AND SHIITAKE MUSHROOMS

****

This is vegan speak for a full fry. Good for lazy evenings and sedate brain cells. Just make sure your tofu is biodynamic and organic to avoid the dodgy mechanical isolation techniques many processors use. (For more on this, see pages 13-14).

Shiitake mushrooms are good for the immune system, according to Dale Pinnock, The Medicinal Chef. Their polysaccharides play funny games with our frontline defenses, resulting in some serious moves against invading pathogens. The herb turmeric has been implicated in the reduction of tumors, amyloid plaque in Alzheimer's, and many other inflammatory conditions, such as arthritis, so we've stuck a good tablespoon in for you. There's raw garlic too, vaunted for its healing powers. Think Pac-Man in your bloodstream. In other words, this is a good dish to have up your sleeve alongside your emergency Kleenex.

1 onion
About 8 shiitake (or other) mushrooms
2 tablespoons extra virgin olive or coconut oil
About 8 cherry tomatoes
Splash of tamari, plus extra to serve
One 14 oz (397 g) block of firm tofu
1 garlic clove, crushed
1 tablespoon ground turmeric
2 teaspoons ground cumin
1 teaspoon nutritional yeast flakes or a pinch of salt
Cayenne pepper, to serve

Serves 3

Slice or dice the onion and shiitakes, depending how you like to eat them. In a warm frying pan, add the oil, onion, mushrooms, and cherry tomatoes and cook for 10 minutes, until the onions turn glassy and translucent. If your frying pan looks overcrowded, watch out. Steam won't escape and will waterlog your breakfast instead of caramelizing it. I like to roast or grill my tomatoes with a lick of balsamic vinegar and olive oil and add them to the mushrooms before plating up. While I find this method best, it does add to the washing up.

Once the onions and mushrooms are cooked, add a splash of tamari and stir briskly as the pan sizzles. This will dress the mushrooms in some finger-licking umami. Add the block of firm tofu and crumble it under a wooden spatula. Let the garlic, turmeric, cumin, and yeast flakes join the party, digging any white pieces of tofu into the bright yellow turmeric glaze. As soon as it's warmed through, serve with cayenne pepper, tamari soy sauce, and some good company.

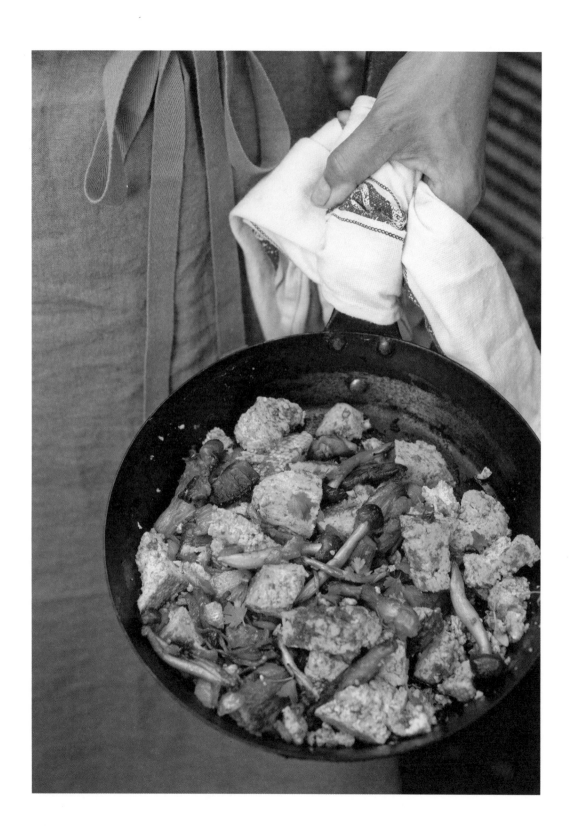

BAKED SWEET POTATOES

****

Ambrosial, warm, and comforting-everything a breakfast should be on a chilly morning. Sweet potatoes are superheroes of the soil. Expect to ramp up your frontline defenses after breakfasting on these. You'll find lots of beta-carotene, zinc, vitamin E, and vitamin C within its amber flesh. These are the nutrients responsible for fancy immune ripostes. Think Catherine Zeta-Jones and Zorro. The sniffles won't stand a chance.

2 medium sweet potatoes
A little time

Serves 1-2

Throw the potatoes into the oven, whole and in their skins. Bake at 400°F (200°C) for 60-90 minutes, depending on their size. There's no need to pierce or slit the potato skins. Sweet potatoes will steam beautifully in their own jackets if you leave them alone. Remove when very soft to touch. Sweet potatoes benefit from overcooking rather than undercooking.

GREEN EGGS

****

Matcha is the Rolls Royce of green teas. The whole tea leaf is ground into a powder, as opposed to diluted in a tea bag. This might help explain why matcha has significantly more antioxidants and pomposity than regular green tea. This neon green powder also houses a gob-smacking amount of protective catechins. Health scientists get indecently excited about these compounds. Be careful not to fall for all the hype of 137 antioxidants per sip, bottomless libido, and eternal life. But it does make scrambled eggs more interesting.

Green eggs take 3 minutes from start to finish. Double up to serve a friend.

Gently warm the coconut oil in a heavy-based pan on medium heat, making sure the oil doesn't reach smoke point. Butter and cream are supposedly the best allies to making the perfect scrambled eggs, but something very special happens when they cavort with coconut oil instead. You're about to find out.

Break the eggs into a bowl and whisk briefly with a fork. Add them to the heated pan and let them cook halfway through before stirring them. I like my eggs luscious and floppy, so I take them off now and plate up. El Hubador prefers his fluffy and seriously scrambled, so I leave his on for a further 10 seconds and stir with a vigor usually reserved for rowing a sinking boat. Stir through the chives or chervil and season once cooked. Whatever way you like yours, just remember not to add the matcha powder until the scrambled eggs are served up. Use a sieve to sprinkle the green powder over them like angel dust.

2 teaspoons extra virgin coconut oil

3 eggs

2 teaspoons chopped chives or chervil

Generous pinch of salt and crushed black peppercorns

$1/4$ teaspoon matcha green tea powder

Serves 1

MISO EGGS AND SOY SAUCE

****

Butter and cream are supposedly the best allies to making the perfect scrambled eggs, but something very special happens when eggs fraternize with coconut oil and miso.

4 teaspoons extra virgin
  coconut oil
5 eggs
2 teaspoons live,
  unpasteurized miso
Splash of tamari

Serves 2

Gently warm the coconut oil in a heavy-based pan on medium heat, making sure the oil doesn't reach smoke point.

Break the eggs into a bowl and whisk briefly with the miso. Add to the heated pan and let the eggs cook halfway through before stirring them. I prefer mine soft and floppy, so I fold the eggs over like an omelette and plate up. If you prefer them cooked for longer, stir briskly until the eggs look fluffy. This usually makes the miso silky smooth as opposed to lumpy.

Whatever way you like yours, just remember not to add the tamari until the scrambled eggs are served up. Otherwise you'll end up with murky-looking eggs, which don't go well with hangovers.

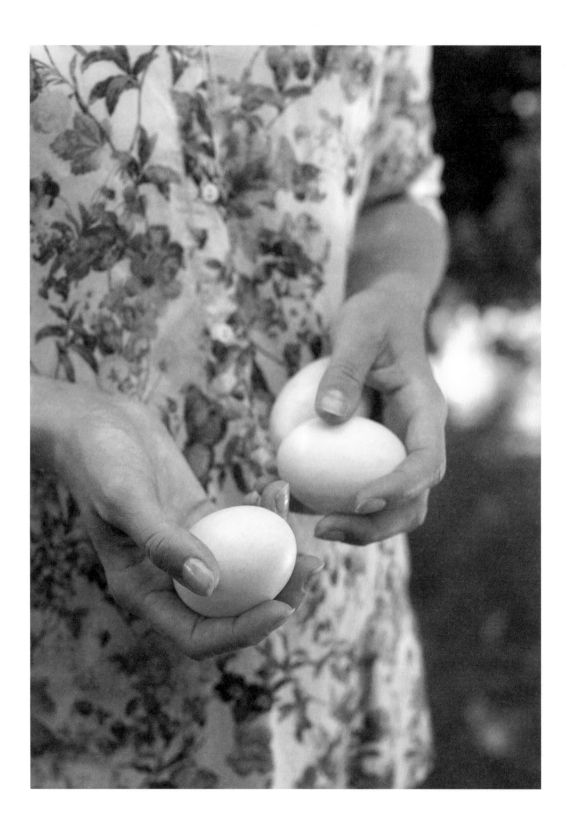

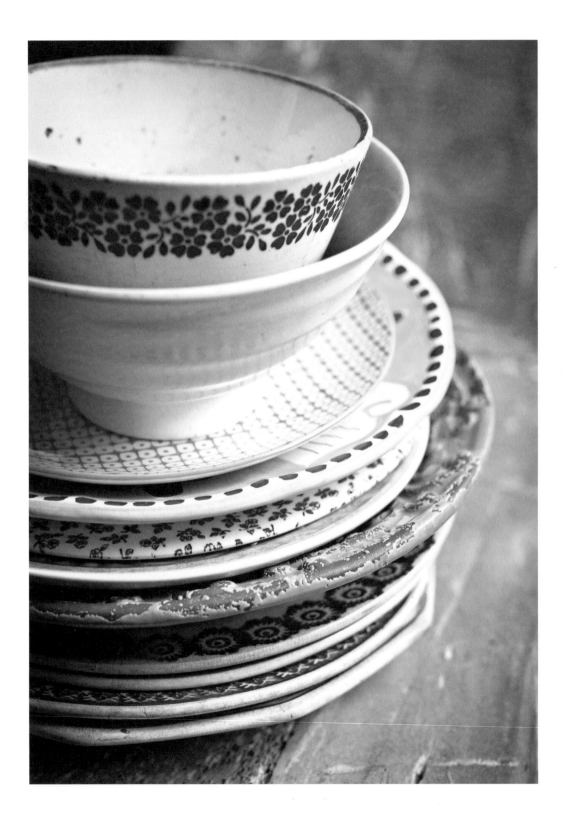

MILLET AND CHESTNUT CRÊPES WITH PASSION FRUIT SYRUP

****

This recipe is borrowed (and butchered) from Béatrice Peltre's award-winning blog, La Tartine Gourmande. Turns out Béa married my mother-in-law's cousin's son. That makes me practically French. Three times removed, of course, but what's a number, right?

Combine the flour, sugar, and salt in a large bowl. The sugar is an important addition, so please do leave it in the recipe. Break the eggs into the center of the flour and slowly whisk while pouring in the milk. Continue to whisk until the batter is silky. Stir in the coconut oil and vanilla. Cover with a plate and place in the fridge to rest for 1 hour, or overnight.

When ready to use, stir again. In a crêpe pan or frying pan, melt a little more coconut oil. Swirl to coat. Add enough batter to barely coat the bottom. You may have to shake the pan a little. Cook for 1–2 minutes on medium to high heat. Once it starts bubbling and the batter looks cooked through, flip the crêpe and cook for 1 extra minute on the other side. Repeat until you run out of batter, adding a little coconut oil between each crêpe. Keep the crêpes warm on a plate as you work, covering them with a towel.

To make the syrup, just combine the pulp of the passion fruit with your choice of sweetener and drizzle over your creations. Homemade apple syrup is like a flavor grenade, so try to give the recipe on page 25 a go.

$^1/_4$ cup (25 g) millet flour
$^1/_2$ cup (65 g) chestnut flour
2 tablespoons cornflour
2 tablespoons rapadura or coconut sugar
Pinch of sea salt
2 eggs
1 cup (250 ml) hemp, oat, or almond milk
1 tablespoon extra virgin coconut oil, melted, plus extra to cook
1 teaspoon pure vanilla extract
2 passion fruit
2 tablespoons raw honey or apple or date syrup

Makes 10 crêpes

SMOKED SALMON BLINI WITH HEALTHIER HOLLANDAISE

****

If you could do one thing to improve your health this year, swap your nasty margarine and commercial salad dressing for this incredibly sumptuous mayonnaise. When made with warm coconut oil, it rivals the most heavenly hollandaise to ever kiss a blini.

For the "hollandaise":
2 egg yolks
$1^1/_4$ cup (60 ml) flaxseed oil
 or Udo's Oil
$^1/_4$ cup (60 ml) extra virgin
 coconut oil, melted
2 big garlic cloves, crushed
1-2 tablespoons unpasteurized
 apple cider vinegar
$^1/_2$ cup (125 ml) extra virgin
 olive oil
6-8 anchovies, roughly
 chopped

For the buckwheat blini:
1 cup (140 g) buckwheat flour
1 teaspoon baking powder
Salt and freshly ground
 black pepper
1 egg
$^2/_3$ cup (165 ml) almond, hemp,
 or oat milk
Extra virgin coconut oil for
 frying
8-10 slices of smoked salmon

Makes 8-10 big blini

To make the "hollandaise," run the motor of your food processor with the egg yolks. Keeping the motor on low, gradually add a steady stream of flaxseed oil and watch it thicken ever so gradually. Add it drop by drop-don't rush or you will end up curdling it, as I have done through impatience and overexcitement many a time. This can take up to 4 minutes. Repeat with the coconut oil. When it gets very thick, it's time to add the crushed garlic and apple cider vinegar to thin it out and give it an edge. Keep the motor running.

Next, slowly add the olive oil, watching the mayo thicken again. Always add the olive oil after the coconut oil and not the other way around. Olive oil can turn bitter if overly whisked.

Finally, add the anchovies and pulse briefly-you don't want to pulverize the anchovies. Taste and adjust the sharpness of the apple cider vinegar to your preference. If it's too sharp, turn on the motor again and add a little more olive oil.

Scoop into a screw-top jar and refrigerate for up to 3 weeks. A jar is approximately 16 portions.

To make the blini, sieve the flour, baking powder, and a generous amount of seasoning into a bowl. In a separate cup, beat the egg with the milk and gradually pour into the dry ingredients, whisking all the while to prevent lumps. The batter lasts for 2 days in the fridge, so advance preparation is easy.

Heat some extra virgin coconut oil in a large nonstick frying pan on medium to high heat. Drop enough of the blini batter to form a drop scone and fry for 20-30 seconds, until set. Several can be done at once. Flip to cook the other side. The mixture is usually runny on one

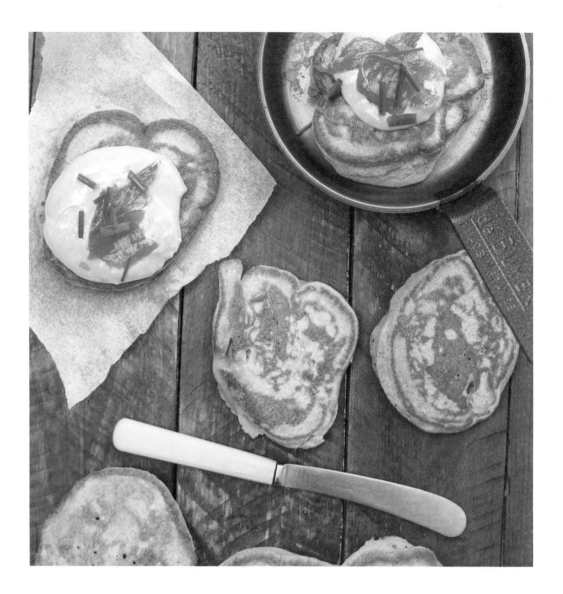

side, so flip with haste. Try not to leave them cooking too long or they will dry out. Taste the first one when cooled and decide for yourself. Hot blini will always taste moist, but they quickly lose their juiciness upon cooling. Bear this in mind too.

Repeat until there is no batter left. Dollop with the hollandaise and a blanket of smoked salmon. Pretty special stuff.

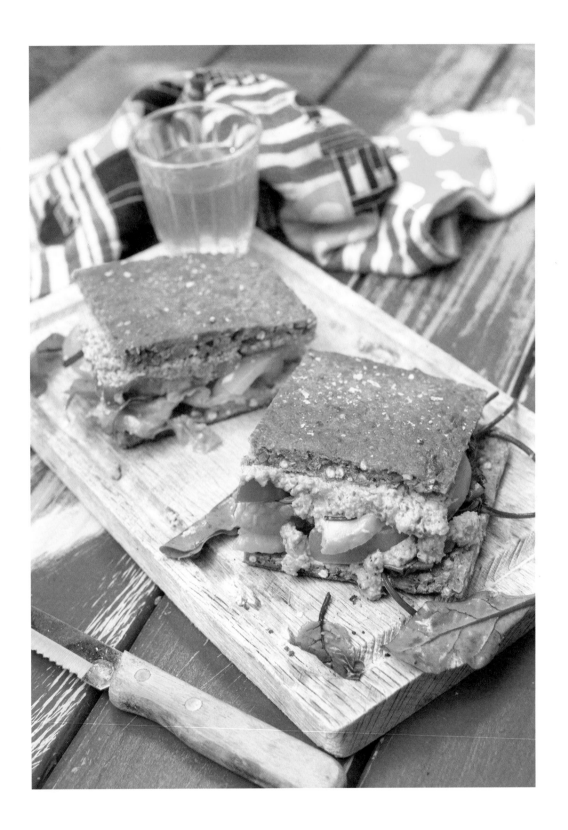

YOUR NEW WHEAT-FREE BREAD

****

Few pleasures in life can compete with loafing into hot soda bread, straight from the oven. I'm not going to suggest you give bread up—that would be bonkers and deeply unnecessary. Food is about joy, not penance.

For a nourishing alternative, I recommend inaugurating this bread to your life. And to your freezer. It tastes like Irish brown bread but without the bloating often associated with factory-made bread. I've included loads of whole-grains to help your synapses do somersaults. Few breads can compete with that!

Preheat the oven to 400°F (200°C). Line a shallow tray just smaller than a magazine page with parchment paper. We're going to bake this in a tray rather than a loaf pan, so when it's cooked, we'll cut it into squares. Each square can be used for a sandwich, sliced horizontally.

Sieve the flours, baking powder, seasoning, and spices into a large bowl to introduce air and make the bread fluffy. Try not to omit the spices, as they are central to this bread. Add the milk, millet flakes, sunflower seeds, whole buckwheat grains, and honey (if using). It should be a pouring consistency and be quite runny. Pour the batter into the lined tray.

Bake for 35–40 minutes, depending on the depth of the tray you are using. Remove from the oven, allow to cool on a wire rack and divide into quarters. Looks really slick. Freeze in quarters, ready to split horizontally and toast every morning.

If your first attempt at this bread felt undercooked, an oven thermometer will canter to the rescue. I bring mine to every kitchen I cook in. You'd be shocked at the number of ovens that lie!

$1/2$ cup (70 g) buckwheat flour
$1/2$ cup (50 g) organic soy flour
2 teaspoons baking powder
1 teaspoon Herbamare seasoning, celery salt, or sea salt
1 teaspoon ground ginger
1 teaspoon ground cinnamon
2 cups (500 ml) almond, oat, or hemp milk
$3/4$ cup (90 g) millet or barley flakes
$3/4$ cup (90 g) sunflower seeds
$1/2$ cup (100 g) whole buckwheat grains
$1/2$ tablespoons honey, barley malt extract, or maple syrup (optional)

Makes 1 loaf

RYE BANANA BREAD WITH HOMEMADE CHOCOLATE HAZELNUT SPREAD

****

This is a crazy delicious vegan banana bread made with one of my favorite whole-grains.

Rye is rich in B vitamins, the chaps that act as spark plugs for energy ignition. This grain is also thought to have a higher concentration of cancer-protective lignans than any other cereal crop. Even more interesting, rye is the grain of choice for bodybuilders because of its specific amino acid profile, which seems to fancy muscle mass. But don't worry-you won't end up looking like a Transformer by nibbling away on this banana bread. You've got to lift insane amounts of weights to do that.

If you're looking for a totally gluten-free recipe, just replace the rye flour with a combination of buckwheat and brown rice flour. Barley malt extract also works well, but honey doesn't, for some strange reason.

For the bread:
1/2 cup (100 g) extra virgin
   coconut oil, butter, or ghee
11/4 cups (170 g) coconut
   sugar
4 (350 g) bananas, mashed
Generous pinch of sea salt
1 tablespoon psyllium husks
1/2 cup natural soy yogurt or
   any plant-based milk
2 teaspoons vanilla extract
11/4 cups (180 g) coarse rye
   flour
2 teaspoons baking powder

For the spread:
1/3 cup (90 g) hazelnut butter
   (about half a small jar)
3 tablespoons cacao or cocoa
   powder
2 tablespoons maple or brown
   rice syrup

Makes 1 loaf

Preheat the oven to 350°F (180°C). You'll need a small to medium loaf pan, lined and ready.

To make the spread, whip the ingredients together in a cup using a fork.

For the banana bread, whiz everything in a food processor.

Scrape into the loaf pan and smooth the top with your tongue or a spoon. Whichever seems preferable.

Once the oven is pre-heated, bake for 1 hour. Remove from the oven and let the banana bread sit in its pan for 10 minutes before delicately removing. Cool on a wire rack or stack of linen. The bread will be ready to slice in 1 hour. Amen.

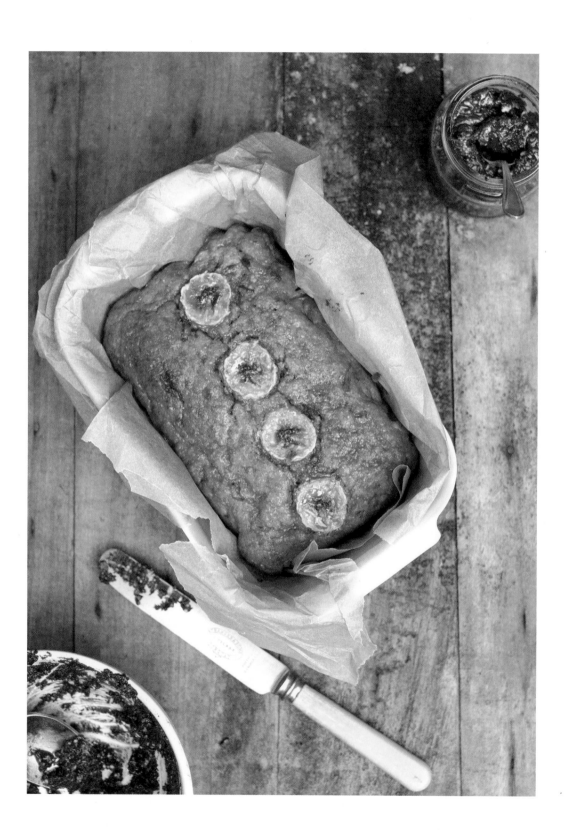

FLAXSEED FOCACCIA WITH OLIVES AND SUN-DRIED TOMATOES

****

Omega-3 oils are to hormones what Dolce is to Gabbana: indispensable. Our bodies cannot make omega-3, so we need to regularly include it in our diet. As always, food sources are preferable to supplements. You'll find a decent supply of omega-3 fatty acids in this bread. Flaxseeds are also said to be one of nature's highest sources of cancer-protective plant lignans. These groovy compounds are linked to happy hormones, lower blood cholesterol, and boisterous antioxidant behavior. Quite the hat trick for a tiny seed.

If you know someone who is gluten intolerant or celiac, please jot this recipe down and gift it to them. It contains no flour or grains, making it perfect for paleo disciples too. But you don't have to be a paleo geek to appreciate this bread—it's incredibly good for you and seriously tasty.

I prefer to use blackstrap molasses instead of honey for three reasons. First, it gives the best baking results. Second, it's superrich in iron and B vitamins for energy. And third, it's much cheaper.

2 cups (220 g) grand flaxseeds
3 teaspoons dried oregano
2 teaspoons baking powder
4 eggs
$^1/_2$ cup (125 ml) hemp or almond
  milk
4 tablespoons extra virgin
  olive or macadamia oil
2 tablespoons blackstrap
  molasses or honey, warmed
  until runny
10–12 small sun-dried or
  sun-blushed tomatoes
Handful of black olives,
  stones removed

Makes 1 loaf

Preheat the oven to 350°F (180°C). Lightly oil or line a small baking tray that's a few inches smaller than an A4 page. Brownie pans are perfect—either an 8 x 8- or a 10 x 8-inch.

Combine the ground flaxseeds, oregano, and baking powder together in a large bowl. Set aside.

In a separate bowl, mix the eggs, milk, oil, and molasses until thoroughly united.

Chop up the sun-dried tomatoes and olives and add them to the wet ingredients. Now add wet to dry and immediately pour into your greased baking tray. Spread evenly and sprinkle a little more dried oregano on top.

Bake for about 25 minutes, then remove from the oven and its pan. Allow to cool for 25 minutes on a wire rack. Tickle with black olive tapenade, some supergarlicky hummus, or serve alongside your favorite bowl of soup. This bread freezes exceptionally well, ready to grill when there's nothing in the cupboard.

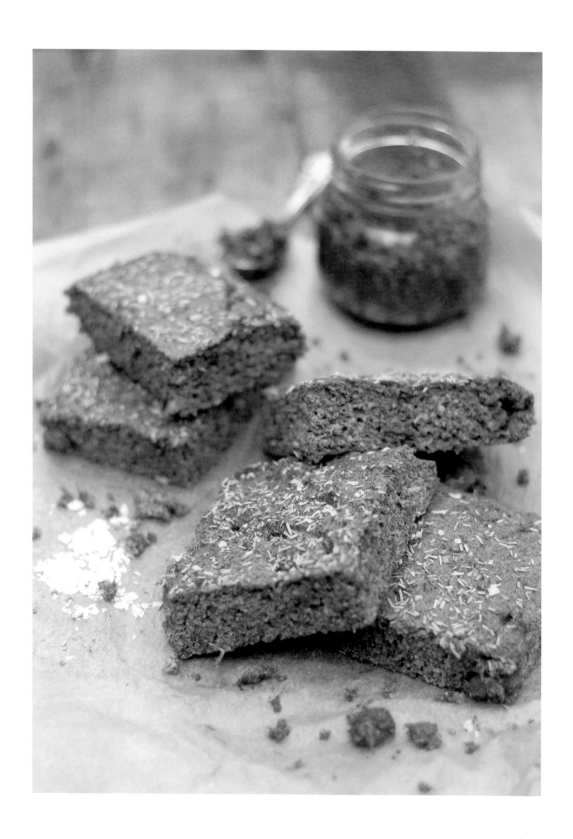

MULTISEED RYE BREAD WITH CARAWAY SPICE

****

Trying to cut down on butter and baguettes? Difficult, isn't it? Now's a good time to create fresh associations with the food you eat in order to break the unhealthy ones.

David A. Kessler has written a gripping book about how junk food hijacks our brain chemistry and controls our behavior. Reading even one chapter of Kessler's The End of Overeating feels so liberating and empowering. Kessler cautions us that certain cues activate brain circuits that guide behavior. Instead of attacking the behavior (overeating, smoking, reaching for more butter, insert vice here), recognize the cue.

For example, can you watch TV without reaching for a snack? Or have a coffee without smoking a cigarette? In other words, it's the cue that needs reformulating if we are to successfully ditch the junk in our diets. It's not enough to put a fatwa on the food. We need to acknowledge the prompts. So what are your cues?

Kessler's advice is to create fresh associations in an attempt to retrain our behavior and palate. I recommend putting caraway and aniseed into your bread. Such a simple change will help keep your mitts off that errant butter dish. Caraway and aniseed are so much tastier when paired with olive oil. Your taste buds will break dance.

3/4 cup (100 g) pumpkin seeds
3/4 cup (90 g) sunflower seeds
3/4 cup (115 g) flaxseeds
1/4 cup (40 g) rapadura or
    coconut sugar
Just under 1¼ cups (300 ml)
    warm water
2 teaspoons fast-action
    organic yeast
Roughly 3 cups (400 g) rye
    flour or 50% rye, 50% white,
    if preferred
2 tablespoons extra virgin
    olive or macadamia oil
1 tablespoon caraway seeds
1 teaspoon sea salt flakes

Makes 1 loaf

Start by lightly toasting the pumpkin and sunflower seeds on a baking tray in the oven for 12 minutes at 350°F (180°C) with no oil. Leave to cool. I recommend toasting more than you need, as hot, crunchy seeds are often looted in my house.

Once cooled, transfer the toasted seeds and flaxseeds into a large mixing bowl with the sugar, warm water and yeast. Let these guys laze for 10 minutes before adding the remaining ingredients. Mix into a firm dough and leave for another 10 minutes.

Now briefly and lightly knead the dough. Leave in the bowl, covered with a clean cloth, for 1 hour in a warm spot. Transfer to a suitable loaf pan lined with parchment paper. You'll need to squish in the sides a little. Cover and leave to rise for about another hour. The time will depend on the type of yeast you have used, so as soon as the dough looks about 20 percent bigger, you're in business.

Bake for 45 minutes at 400°F (200°C). Remove from the
oven and from its pan and cool on a wire rack. Best
sliced thinly.

You'll love this multiseed bread. It tastes incredible
warm from the oven, but you can gently toast some slices
the next day to achieve similar results. For a funky
change, add a teaspoon of ground fenugreek, aniseed, and
fennel seeds.

Snacks and Other Nutritional Hits

"Health is beauty. If someone takes care of themselves,
you can see the health shining from within them."
—Anna Friel, actress

The definition of madness is doing the same thing over
and over again but expecting different results. If your body
isn't functioning as well as you'd like it to, take a
look at what you're putting into it. Eating foods that
promote good health will have you on your tippy toes.
Eating foods that promote poor health will have you on your
knees. It's as simple as that.

Many of these snacks can be stored in the freezer, lined up
like soldiers for when the munchies attack. This is an
important feature of a good, wholesome diet. If you don't
have back-up, you're sure to fall under enemy fire.

Of course, there will be occasions when we
fraternize with the enemy (insert vice here).
No matter. Move on and try a few of these recipes
to get yourself back on track.

HOT AND SMOKY SEEDS

+++++++++++++++++++++++++++++

Touche Éclat and espressos must be keeping our economy afloat. Over half of us reportedly suffer from some sort of sleep disorder. So when it comes to nodding off, what are the smarter options? If self-hypnosis and chamomile tea never worked for you, take a close look at your diet and see if you are getting enough B vitamins (especially B6), zinc, and the amino acid L-tryptophan.

Foods rich in tryptophan can be an effective sleep aid without you having to subscribe to dodgy narcotics. Tryptophan is the building block for an important snoozy hormone called melatonin. Without it, our eyes will struggle to shut.

Here's the good news. You'll find tryptophan, B vitamins, and zinc in pumpkin seeds. As a result, scientists have begun to put pumpkin seed extract in multivitamin pills and sleeping aids. Bear in mind that it's easier and cheaper to keep a stash of pumpkin seeds in your fridge. But don't expect to fall straight to sleep if you eat them. Think of pumpkin seeds as couriers, delivering the cargo your body needs later tonight.

Roughly 1¹/₂ cups (200 g)
   combination of pumpkin and
   sunflower seeds
2 tablespoons tamari
1 tablespoon mirin (optional)
1 teaspoon dried chili flakes
1 tablespoon dried nori flakes
   (optional calcium boost)

Makes 1¹/₂ cups

Preheat the oven to 350°F (180°C).

Toss the sunflower and pumpkin seeds on a baking tray and roast for 8-10 minutes. Now it's time to add the tamari, mirin, and chili flakes. Coat well, using a wooden spatula to stir the seeds about so as not to scrape your tray. Return to the oven for an extra 1-2 minutes of toasting.

Remove from the oven to cool and stir through the nori flakes (if using). Shards of Crispy Kale (page 63) also work. Once cooled, the seeds become crunchy again. Refrigerate in a screw-top jar and sprinkle over salads and soups or keep a stash in your pocket. They can last for up to 6 weeks.

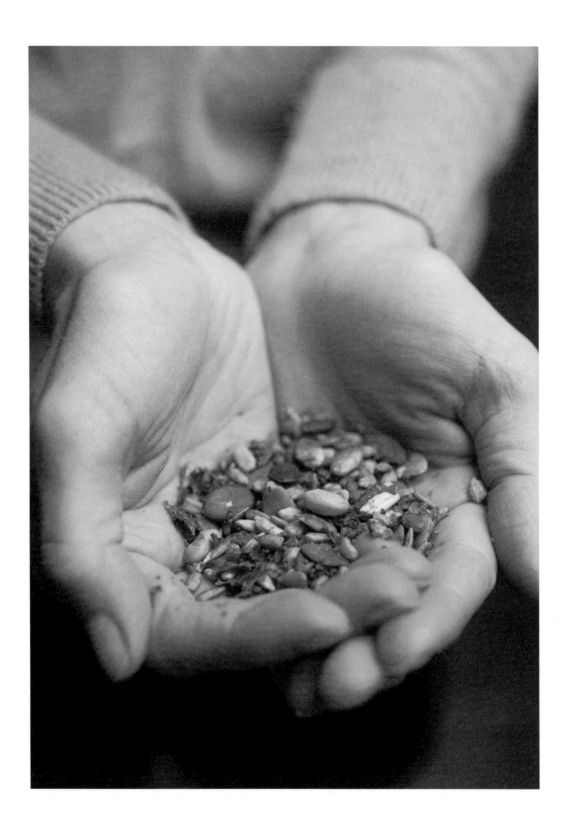

OFFICE BOMBS

++++++++++++++

Office Bombs love lunchboxes, gym bunnies, and little mitts. They take just minutes to prepare, but the benefits last all day. These snacks are designed to drip-feed your battery consistently instead of giving you one big sugar surge. Perfect fodder to help high-jump that 3 o'clock afternoon trap.

If you can't find the large packets of ground sunflower and pumpkin seeds, just whiz enough of both seeds until they resemble fine breadcrumbs.

2 tea bags of raspberry leaf
  tea, opened
2 cups (240 g) combination of
  ground pumpkin and sunflower
  seeds
1 cup (150 g) raisins, chopped
1/2 cup (45 g) ground almonds
  (or more ground seeds)
1/2 cup (125 ml) tahini
1/2 cup (125 ml) honey, or
  maple or brown rice syrup
4 tablespoons raw cacao nibs
5 tablespoons carob powder
Pinch of good-quality salt,
  like pink Himalayan
Desiccated coconut, to coat

Makes 30

Blitz everything except the desiccated coconut in your food processor just long enough for the mixture to start clumping together. You may need to scrape down the sides as you go along. Alternatively, with the assistance of some tunes and tenacity, beat the ingredients together with a simple metal fork.

Roll the dough between your palms into golf ball-size treats. Drop them into a bowl of desiccated coconut to turn them into Office Bombs. They'll keep for 3 weeks in the fridge, 3 months in the freezer, or 3 seconds in your hands.

CRISPY KALE

++++++++++++++

I experimented with nineteen batches of kale chips and over forty guinea piglets. My taste buds had to be validated. After all, kale is a green leafy vegetable, the kind that tends to repel even the intrepid herbivores among us. Suddenly it was casting a spell upon rambling little fingers.

Not one of my guinea piglets gagged when I divulged the core ingredient. A couple of gasps could be heard, and a few silent screams. The under-tens thought these "chips" were a really naughty snack. One plate later, they had wolfed down more greens than they had in the entire week.

There are a couple of variations you could try. Below is the most basic. Nutritional yeast flakes have an umami buzz. It's cheese to vegans, and replete with that elusive vitamin B12. If your local health food store is out of yeast flakes, use garlic granules and smoked paprika instead.

Preheat the oven to 350°F (180°C).

Flatten the kale leaves and use the point of a knife to remove the tough center ribs. Tear the leaves into bite-size pieces.

Using your hands, massage oil into each leaf. Spread across a baking tray. Don't worry about flattening the leaves out; they're better bunched up. Bake for 8–12 minutes. Check after 6 minutes and toss to prevent charring.

Grind the yeast flakes into a powder using a pestle and mortar. Remove from the oven and sprinkle the powdered yeast over the now-crispy kale. Scoff while warm. I'm not sure if crispy kale keeps in a sealed container. It never gets that far in my house. Also awesome with sweet brown rice, avocado, and tamari for a swift supper.

2 good handfuls of bone-dry
  curly kale
1/2 tablespoon extra virgin
  olive or coconut oil
1 tablespoon nutritional
  yeast flakes

Serves 4

CHIA BONBONS

++++++++++++++++

Chia seeds are an easy way to get those much-coveted omega-3 fats without having to neck back flax oil or pharma bullets.

What's so snazzy about omega-3s? A deficit in omega-3 fats has been linked to angry skin conditions, poor concentration levels, and delinquent hormones. Without omega-3s, it seems we manufacture substandard cells. Not an attractive proposition. Think gazelle or tortoise: which would you rather be?

So will taking omega-3 fats cure mental atrophy, PMS, and sagging boobs? No, but strong evidence suggests it can help. That's enough.

It's worth noting that the type of omega-3 fatty acids found in chia is slightly different to those found in oily fish. Chia contains ALA, the precursor to EPA and DHA fatty acids. You've probably come across these confusing terms at the pharmacy when choosing omega-3 supplements. In short, it has been argued that EPA and DHA are easier for the body to absorb. As a result, the omega-3s present in oily fish like mackerel are thought to be superior to those found in plants such as chia and flax. But chia offers a suite of other goodies, including more calcium than milk, banks of potassium, bone-building boron, and cholesterol-reducing fiber.

4 tablespoons tahini
Nearly $^1/_4$ cup (60 ml) maple
   syrup
$^1/_2$ cup (45 g) ground chia
   seeds
$^1/_4$ cup (25 g) ground almonds
2 tablespoons cocoa or raw
   cacao powder
5 tablespoons desiccated
   coconut

Makes about 30 bonbons

Beat the tahini and syrup together with a fork. Please note that honey won't work in this recipe. Once the tahini mixture is all glossy and luscious, measure in the chia seeds, ground almonds, and cocoa powder and encourage them to party. A wooden spoon is useful.

Put the coconut in a bowl or shallow plate. Roll a small cherry-size ball of mixture between the palms of your hands to form a bonbon. Drop each one into the coconut and roll it around to coat, then let it set on a cold plate. You could try different coatings, like beetroot powder, lúcuma powder, or ground hazelnuts. Store in the fridge and plunder at will.

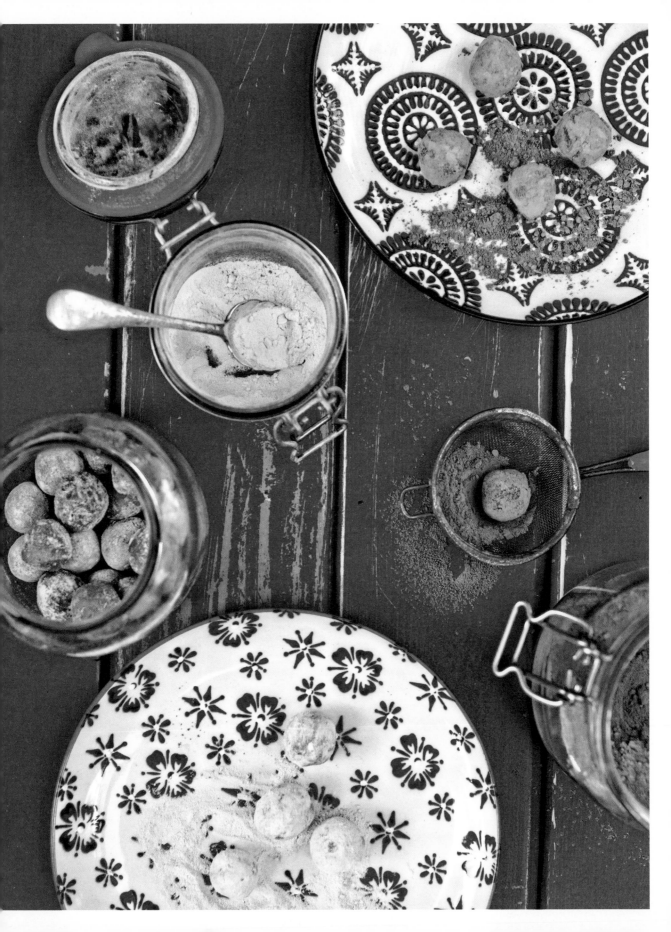

BARLEY GRASS BALLS

+++++++++++++++++++++++

Instead of those dodgy energy drinks, make a big batch of these and store them in the office fridge.

Barley grass is like a mini farm of nutrients. Is it exceptionally rich in any one nutrient? No, but its broad nutritional spectrum makes it a first-rate tonic for dull days. I suspect that eating profuse quantities of green leafy vegetables would offer similar results. Let's agree that barley grass is a lot quicker and easier to prepare.

4 tablespoons ground almonds
4 tablespoons ground pumpkin
  and sunflower seed combo
2 tablespoons tahini
1-2 tablespoons runny honey
1-2 tablespoons barley grass
  powder
Sprinkle of goji berries
  (optional)

Makes about 16 big bonbons

Mush everything together with a fork until it looks like thick cookie dough. Roll a teaspoon of the mixture into little bonbons between your palms. Store in an airtight jar in the fridge and liberate when required.

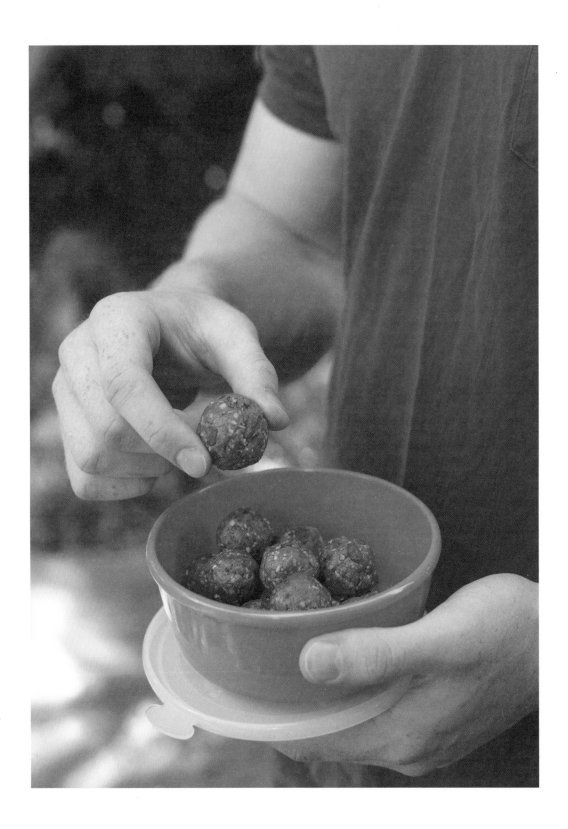

DR. SMOOTHIE

++++++++++++++++

Here's an easy way to start the day with a halo on your head. It doesn't involve broccoli, Lycra, or resetting your alarm clock. Just fruit, live yogurt, oats, and an appetite. OK, and maybe a sense of humor if you forget to put the lid on the blender.

1 very ripe banana or avocado
1 cup frozen berries
1 cup (250 ml) plant milk
$1/2$ cup (125 ml) organic live
  soy or coconut yogurt
4 tablespoons oat flakes
1 tablespoon ground chia or
  flaxseeds

Serves 2-3

The joy of this recipe is that you don't need a special juicer, just your magical whizzy machine. Blend everything together and leave for 1 hour or overnight before scoffing. Bring Dr. Smoothie into work in a jam jar, or savor it on the road when your nerves begin to fray in the bumper-to-bumper traffic. Harness its happiness and you'll be surprised how mellow you'll feel by 8 a.m.

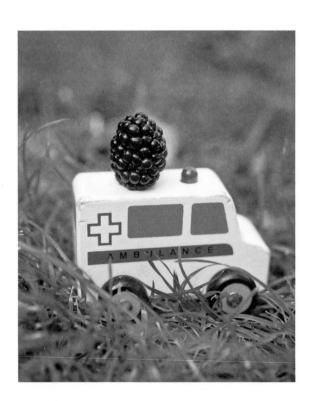

PROTEIN GRENADES

++++++++++++++++++++

These grenades will save you money, fuel your muscles, and feed insatiable appetites. More important, they're much tastier than the commercial sports muck at supermarkets and specialist sports stores.

Hemp protein powder is outrageously tasty, and legal. It comes directly from the hemp plant and contains all eight essential amino acids as well as a nice dose of omega-3 and iron. Iron is responsible for making hemoglobin, which transports oxygen around the blood. No iron, no energy. Omega-3s are important post-training, as they help quench inflammatory markers and heal bruised tissue.

And finally, a word on flaxseeds. They help your pipes. A lot. And offer another round of omega-3 artillery.

Not bad for a bonbon.

Using a fork, mush everything together in a bowl. (Sunwarrior's vegan protein powder is awesome, but it may dent your bank account.)

Roll into mini bonbons and maybe coat each protein grenade with more desiccated coconut. Store in the refrigerator, preferably behind the vegetables, where your housemates will never find them.

2 tablespoons crunchy peanut butter
1 tablespoon hemp seed (protein) powder
1 tablespoon pea protein powder
1 tablespoon ground flaxseeds
1 tablespoon desiccated coconut
1 tablespoon raw agave nectar, honey, or maple syrup
1 tablespoon goji berries (optional)

Makes 8

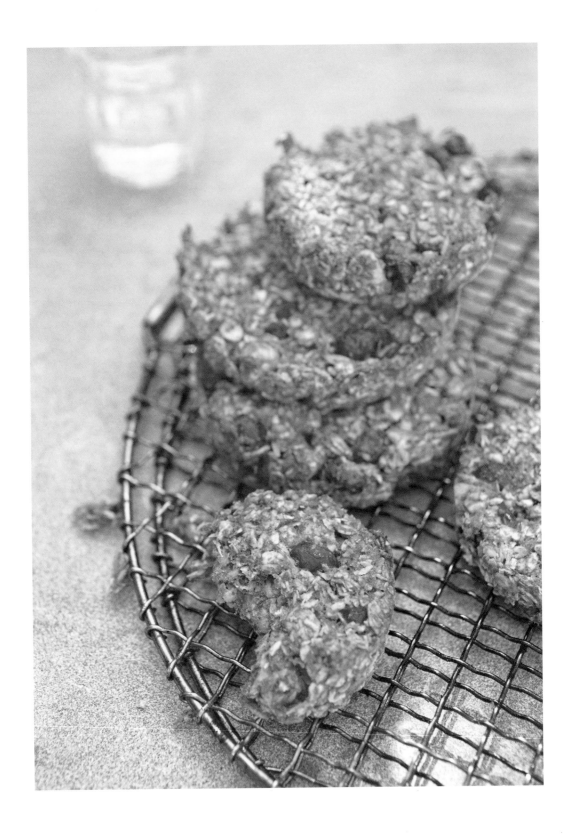

APPLESAUCE AND CINNAMON COOKIES

++

Satisfying and chewy, these are designed as everyday cookies, the sort you sneak into tedious boardrooms.

Raisins are pumped with resveratrol, which acts as a free radical assassin. Free radicals cause damage to our skin and to our arteries by helping LDL cholesterol set up home. Nasty things.

Preheat the oven to 350°F (180°C). Line a large baking tray with parchment paper.

Chop the apples into bite-size chunks and place in a small saucepan with $\frac{1}{4}$ cup of water and your dates or prunes. Cover with a tight-fitting lid and boil for 15 minutes, being careful the apples don't stick to the bottom of the pan. Once the fruit is soft enough to mush, remove from the heat and blitz with a hand-held blender. Measure out $\frac{2}{3}$ cup and set aside. Any leftover purée can be frozen for the next batch of cookies or served on top of yogurt.

Next, finely chop the roasted hazelnuts. There's little point buying pre-chopped hazelnuts, as their good oils turn rancid much quicker. In a large bowl, stir together the chopped hazelnuts, oats, raisins, coconut, flaxseeds, and cinnamon. In a smaller bowl, beat the fruit purée and nut butter together thoroughly, followed by the milk and vanilla. Fold this glossy batter into the dry ingredients and mix thoroughly.

Place a large cookie cutter on the paper-lined tray and spoon the dough into the cookie cutter, filling until it's at least $\frac{3}{4}$ inches deep. Press and smooth with the back of the spoon. Gently lift the cookie cutter up and repeat with the rest of the dough.

Bake for 30 minutes, before they turn brown. Remove from the oven and cool on a wire rack. They can be eaten right away if, like me, you don't have the willpower to wait.

2-3 apples
8 dates or prunes, destoned
4 tablespoons roasted hazelnuts
$1\frac{3}{4}$ cup (160 g) jumbo oat flakes
$\frac{3}{4}$ cup (115 g) raisins and/or dried cranberries
$\frac{3}{4}$ cup (60 g) desiccated coconut
2 tablespoons ground flaxseeds or ground chia seeds
1 tablespoon ground cinnamon
$\frac{1}{4}$ cup (65 g) nut butter, like hazelnut, almond, or macadamia
1 cup (250 ml) organic soy yogurt, or almond, or hemp milk
2 teaspoons vanilla extract

Makes about 12 big cookies

SPIRULINA SHOTS

++++++++++++++++++++

Ever heard of an algae called spirulina? It smells a bit like fermented horse urine. This is usually overlooked once its magic starts to kick in. A favorite among ambitious models, spirulina offers a shortcut to cleansing the body. This curious green powder is home to immodest amounts of protein, calcium, zinc, iron, essential fats, and energy-releasing B vitamins. Spirulina is hailed for helping with everything from lazy limbs to waning libidos.

Manufacturers recommend adding spirulina to yogurts or smoothies. Here's a better way to shoot it back without assaulting your senses, or the kitchen floor.

1 cup unsweetened or fresh
  apple juice
2 teaspoons spirulina powder

Serves 1

Spirulina powder clings to the bottom of cups, so I recommend pouring half the juice into a cup, followed by the spirulina, then the remaining juice. Whisk with a fork. No need to hold your nose-it's surprisingly nice. Or perhaps I'm still asleep when I knock it back.

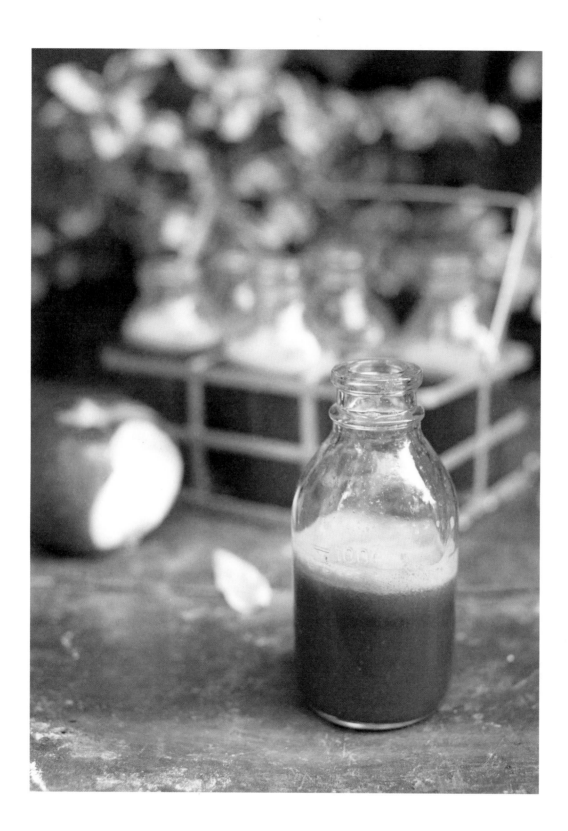

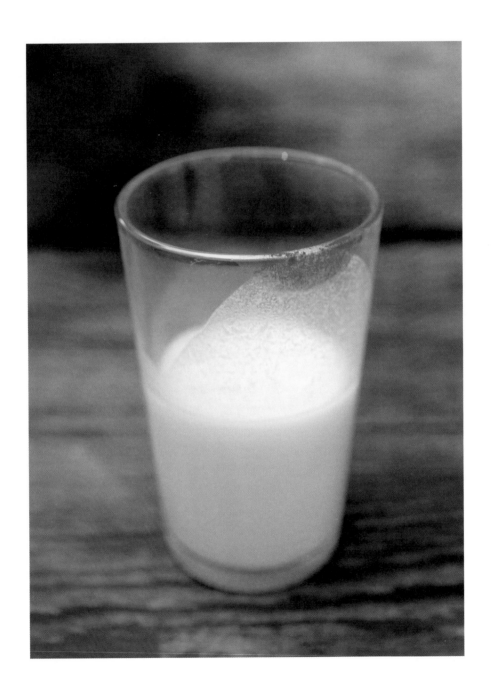

NUT MILK

++++++++++

Brazil nut milk is gorgeous. A Vitamix is the ultimate accessory when making it—and a clean muslin from Mothercare. Since I don't have a Vitamix, my kitchen walls are regularly redecorated. It hasn't stopped me from making nut milk every other week. I drink the milk straightaway or soak muesli in it overnight.

Start by soaking the Brazil nuts overnight or for 24 hours. Rinse and drain. Add 4 fresh cups (750-1000 ml) of water to your Vitamix or food processor along with the vanilla and blitz until silky smooth. In theory, you could add a drop of maple syrup, but I don't think it needs it.

Pour this messy lot into a large jug, using the muslin cloth as a strainer to catch the shards of nuts. A very fine sieve also works. That's it.

1 cup (140 g) Brazil nuts
$1/2$ teaspoon vanilla extract
  or powder (optional)

Makes 1 liter

STRAWBERRY AND BANANA SHOELACES

+++

These popular children's snacks are also called fruit leathers and are usually pumped with sugar and preservatives. DIY versions are easy to make and noticeably tastier. The downside is that they take 6 hours to slow cook. The upside? A strawberry-scented house!

2 cups (330 g) strawberries,
  stems removed
1 banana
1 tablespoon ground flaxseeds
  or ground chia seeds

Makes 15 shoelaces

Blitz all the ingredients in a powerful blender until smooth and glossy. If your strawberries are not fully ripe, you may need to add 1 tablespoon of honey to compensate for any bitterness. I also tried an apple and strawberry combo, which didn't work so well. Looks like banana might be key.

Line a jelly roll pan (a roasting tray with a lip) with parchment paper. Spread the banana and strawberry mix evenly over the parchment with a spatula, making sure it's as smooth as smooth can be. This is the most important step.

If you are lucky enough to own a dehydrator, use your Teflex tray and dehydrate at 108°F (42°C) for 5-6 hours. I use my oven at 140°F (60°C). Depending on the thickness (1/5 inch is perfect), I cook it for 6–8 hours. You will know when it is done-touch and see whether it is still tacky. Remove from the oven once it feels dry to the touch. Allow to cool on the parchment before cutting into shoelaces with scissors, paper and all. The parchment can be removed straightaway or later, when the kiddies attack them.

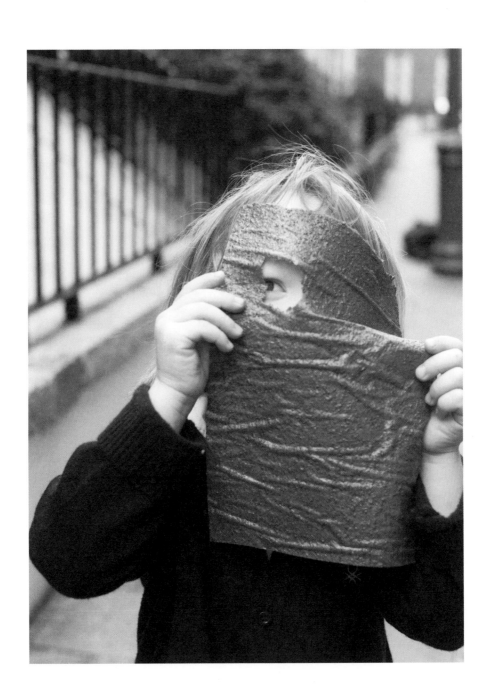

BUCKWHEAT PANCAKES

++++++++++++++++++++++++

Buckwheat pancakes taste sweeter and more wholesome than regular pancakes and are unquestionably more interesting. White flour is nutritionally bland in comparison.

If you're a fan of Japanese take-out, chances are you've already tasted buckwheat in the form of soba noodles. Buckwheat, despite its name, is not wheat at all. It appears to be a relative of rhubarb and is entirely gluten-free.

Russians make blini from buckwheat flour (see page 48) and smother them in caviar for a morning snack. Certainly beats a Kit Kat.

1 cup (140 g) buckwheat flour
Generous pinch of seasoning,
  like Herbamare
2 cups (500 ml) water
Extra virgin coconut oil,
  for frying
1 egg, optional

Makes nine 8-inch pancakes

Stir the flour and seasoning together in a deep jug. Add a little of the water until it forms a smooth paste. Add the remaining water and the optional egg, if using, and whisk, ensuring no lumps appear. Leave to settle for at least 20 minutes or overnight. This makes flipping the pancake much easier when you go to cook the batter.

Heat your non-stick frying pan (non-stick is essential) with $1/2$ tablespoon of coconut oil for each pancake. Using a soup ladle, pour just enough batter onto your hot pan to coat the whole surface. Too much batter will make the pancake too thick to flip. You may need to tilt the pan to cover the whole surface with the batter.

Flip when the underside is cooked. A few practice shots are generally necessary-this is pretty common, so don't beat yourself up over it. The added bonus is munching the unsuccessful ones! By the third or fourth pancake, your results will be flawless.

While the other side of the pancake is cooking, go make yourself some scrambled eggs as a filling. Serve on top of a buckwheat pancake and roll up like a wrap. Any leftover pancakes can be used as cold wraps for lunch at school or the office tomorrow. Try boiling baby potatoes and stirring through crunchy peanut butter, crushing a few spuds along the way to help create a softer filling. A couple of torn salad leaves or fresh cilantro will make it look like you hired Gordon Ramsay to make your lunch.

SUPERFOOD SPREADS - BRAZIL NUT RED PESTO

++

Traditionally, a pesto is made by crushing ingredients into a smooth paste. We're speeding things up here with a cheat's version. The addition of anchovies provides omega-3 oils to our diet as well as boosts brain power with its DMAE phospholipid content. DMAE is believed to convert into the brain nutrient choline, which is useful for remembering important things like the boss's dog's name or where you parked the cursed car. Pregnant mothers feeding on choline-rich foods can also raise their baby's chances of becoming the next president of Mensa.

Throw all the ingredients into a food processor and pulse until the mixure is nicely chopped up and chunky. If the tomatoes were jarred, you won't need additional olive oil. Refrigerate in a screw-top jar until ready to ravage.

12 sun-dried tomatoes
One 2 oz (50 g) can of
 anchovies
Handful of Brazil nuts
Drizzle of extra virgin
 olive oil

Makes 5 portions

SUPERFOOD SPREADS - DIBIS W'RASHI

+++

This is an Iraqi dish that children love to eat with smashed banana or bread. You can make your own date paste by boiling the fruit in a little water for 15 minutes, then whiz until sumptuously smooth.

Whip the tahini and date syrup together with a fork. Add a spot of sea salt if it's not going to find your toddler's mouth. This is good enough to eat straight from a spoon. If stored in a jar in the fridge, this dip will keep for 2 weeks.

4 tablespoons tahini
2 tablespoons date syrup
 or homemade date paste
 (see note above)
Pinch of sea salt

Makes 6 portions

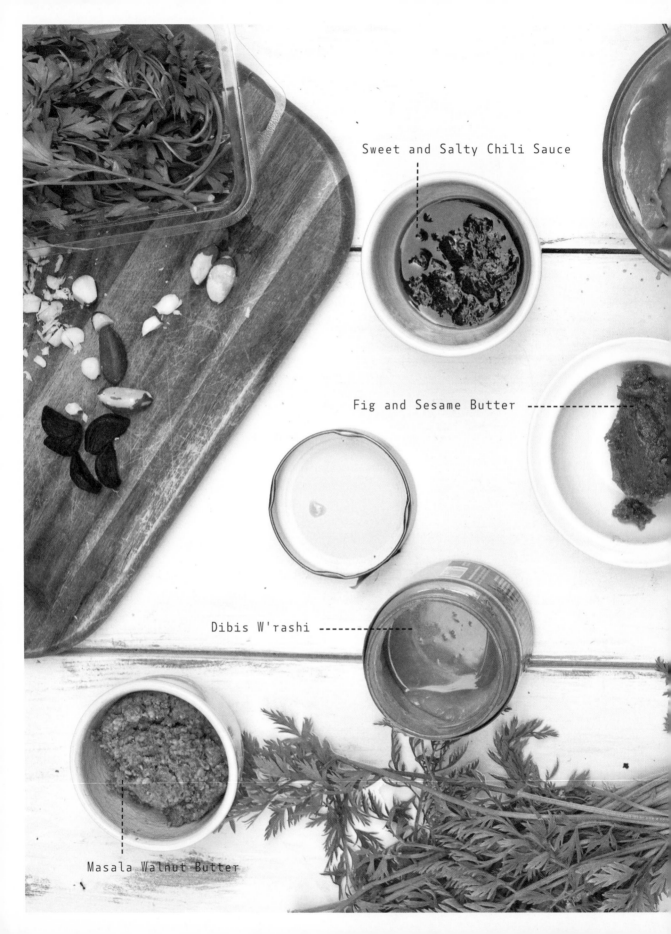

Sweet and Salty Chili Sauce

Fig and Sesame Butter

Dibis W'rashi

Masala Walnut Butter

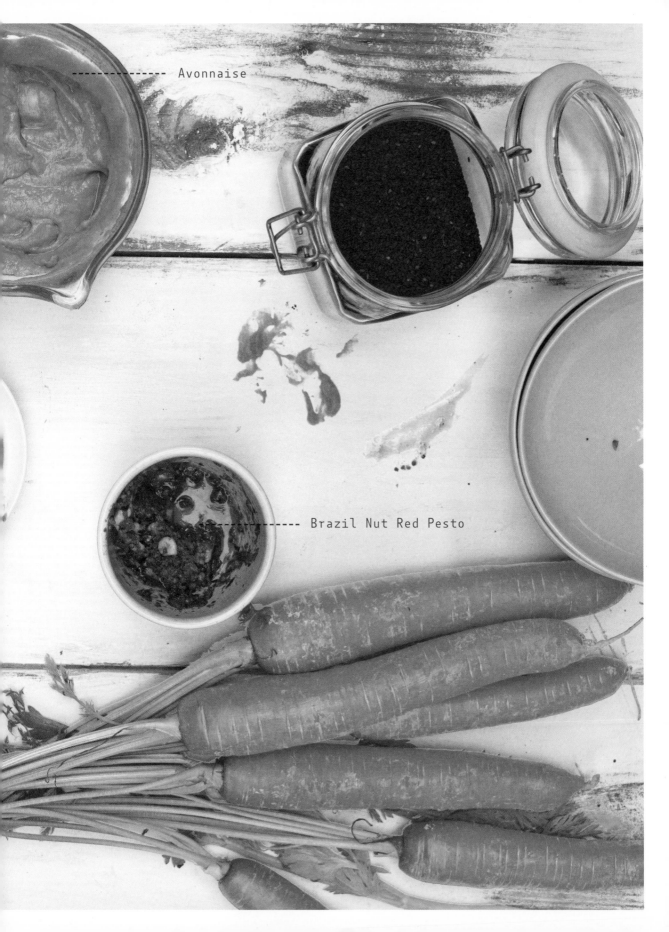

Avonnaise

Brazil Nut Red Pesto

SUPERFOOD SPREADS - MASALA WALNUT BUTTER

+++

When pounded to a pulp with a pestle and mortar, walnuts' natural omega oils are released and meld together to make a decadent butter, heaps healthier than the dairy equivalent. While it's true that walnuts are made up of approximately 60 percent fat, their natural omega-3 oils power your brain, not your waistline.

Look out for stale or oxidized walnuts. They're about as bitter as Simon Cowell. Try to keep walnuts in the fridge and source from reputable stores with a high turnover.

1 good mugful (150 g) of
   walnuts
1 garlic clove
1 teaspoon garam masala
Sprinkle of sea salt flakes
1 teaspoon lemon juice
Raw carrots, cucumbers, or
   bell peppers, as dippers

Makes 5 portions

Break up the walnuts and add to your trusty mortar alongside the garlic, garam masala, and salt. Pound for about 5 minutes with a pestle, until you've got an oily butter. If it's still crumbly, keep on going.

Add 1 tablespoon of water and the lemon juice. Water tends to change the color of the mixture from biscuity brown to light beige. Don't worry-you're on the right track. It's really up to you how creamy or thick you want it. As a guide, 2 tablespoons of water should be ample. Taste and decide if you'd like more spice or crushed garlic.

Dig in using strips of carrot, cucumber, or bell pepper. As a starter for a dinner party, you can make great pass-aroundies by filling a teeny Brussels sprout leaf with this spread and crowning it with a juicy red currant.

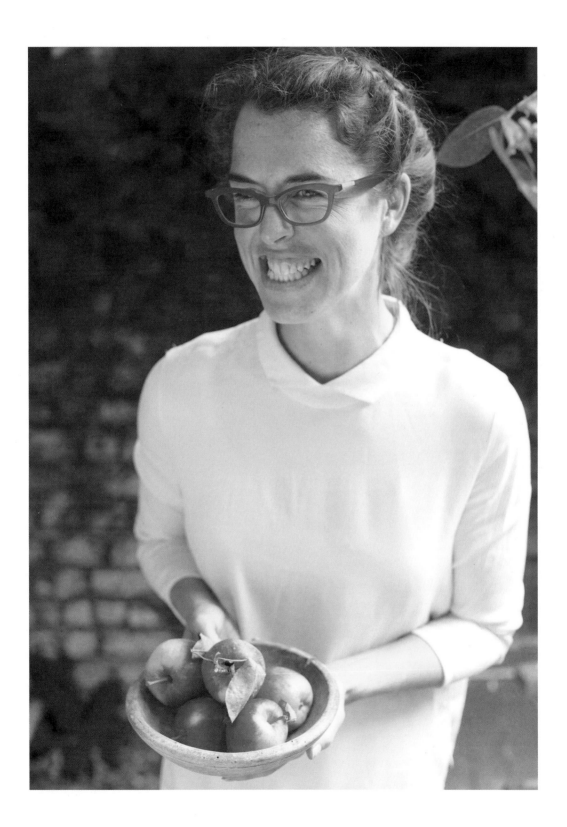

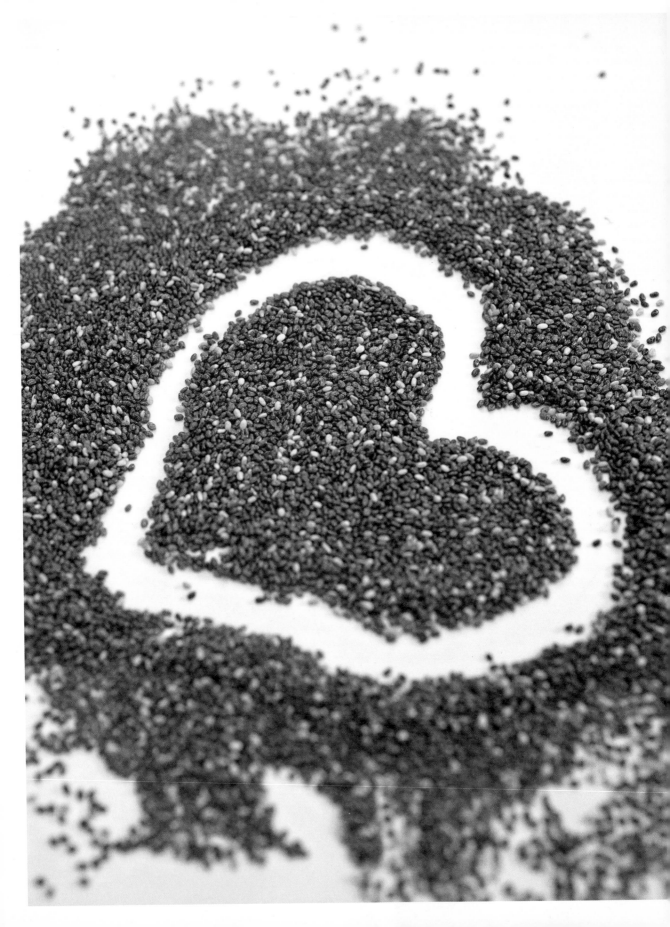

SUPERFOOD SPREADS - OMEGA PARSLEY BUTTER

+++

Think about it-your skin is made from the inside, not the outside. This recipe specifically combines pumpkin seeds' rich source of zinc, lemon's vitamin C, hemp's protein, the essential omega fats from seeds, and parsley's stock of chlorophyll. In other words, it's a real beauty bullet.

Mince the garlic, or grate it with the teeny-tiny part of your grater. Follow with the lemon rind, then squeeze its juice. Give everything a jolly good whiz in the blender until smooth. Store in a scrupulously clean jam jar, with an extra drizzle of olive oil on top. In theory, it should keep for 2 weeks in the fridge. In practice, well, that's another thing. Supertasty on avocados, crackers, sliced cucumber, tomato, bread sticks, or Sunday's roast chicken.

1 small garlic clove
$1/2$ unwaxed lemon
1 bunch of parsley, finely chopped
3 tablespoons hemp seeds
3 tablespoons pumpkin seeds
2 tablespoons extra virgin olive oil
1 tablespoon hemp or flaxseed oil
1 tablespoon sunflower seeds
$1/2$ teaspoon good-quality sea salt

Makes 6 portions

SUPERFOOD SPREADS - FIG AND SESAME BUTTER

+++

Great source of calcium, iron, and finger-licking fun. Oh, and beautiful bowels. My little ones take it to nursery in place of peanut butter.

Remove any stalks from the dried figs, then whiz all the ingredients together in a food processor. Add 1-2 tablespoons of water if you fancy a softer finish. Water won't thin out the spread, but rather will reduce its richness.

Regrigerate in a screw-top jar until ready to ravage.

6 dried figs, soaked overnight
4 tablespoons raw tahini
1-2 tablespoons honey or maple syrup (optional)

Makes 6-8 portions

SUPERFOOD SPREADS - SWEET AND SALTY CHILI SAUCE

++

This is a smashing dip for chicken wings and dunky thangs.

2-3 tablespoons barley malt
  extract, raw agave nectar,
  or yacón syrup
2 tablespoons fresh miso
  paste
2 tablespoons cold-pressed
  toasted sesame oil
$^1/_2$ teaspoon cayenne pepper

Makes 5-6 portions

Whip the ingredients together in a cup with a fork. Serve in a soup bowl to facilitate easy dunking. Leftovers can be stored for 1 week in the fridge.

SUPERFOOD SPREADS - AVONNAISE

++

Fairly deadly with canned tuna, raw carrots, and flax crackers. I love using Herbamare veggie salt in this, from the Swiss naturopath Alfred Vogel. Find it in most good health food shops.

1 large ripe avocado
2-3 tablespoons water
1 teaspoon lemon juice or
  cider vinegar
Black pepper, to taste
Celery salt, to taste

Makes 2 portions

Purée all the ingredients together. You'll need to use a hand-held blender to achieve a super-smooth consistency, like mayonnaise. Taste and adjust the seasoning to your preference. Eat straightaway, as avocados tend to discolor quickly.

SUPERFOOD SPREADS - HOMEMADE CHOCOLATE HAZELNUT SPREAD

++

Makes a great gift for someone feeling poorly.

Whip the ingredients together in a cup using a fork. If you're not planning to eat this DIY Nutella straight away, you can refrigerate it in a clean jam jar for up to 3 weeks. Once chilled, it can be difficult to spread, so add a teaspoon of hot water and beat the Nutella until it's glossy again.

$^{1}/_{3}$ cup (90 g) hazelnut butter (about half a small jar)
3 tablespoons cacao, cocoa, or carob powder
2 tablespoons maple syrup

Makes 6 portions

SUPERFOOD SPREADS - PEANUT BUTTER, BANANA, AND MAPLE SPREAD

++

I usually sneak leftover beans into the mix when I have them. My son is none the wiser, but his bowels certainly are.

Mash all the ingredients together and serve on crackers. This spread is best scoffed right away, as the mashed banana starts to darken with oxidation.

1 ripe banana
2 tablespoons pure peanut butter
Drop of maple syrup
Crackers, to serve

Serves 2-4

Soups

"It's better to pay the grocer than the doctor."
—Michael Pollan

Soups are magical potions. They can resuscitate flat batteries and
pump life through our bodies faster than a voodoo drum.
There's something special about slurping a hot bowl of sunshine and
feeling your veins ignite. When food is in liquid form,
we not only digest it rapidly, we also absorb nutrients
much quicker. Here are some of my favorite recipes to get
your toes tingling. No need for cream, butter, or flour-just
a little love and a wooden spoon.

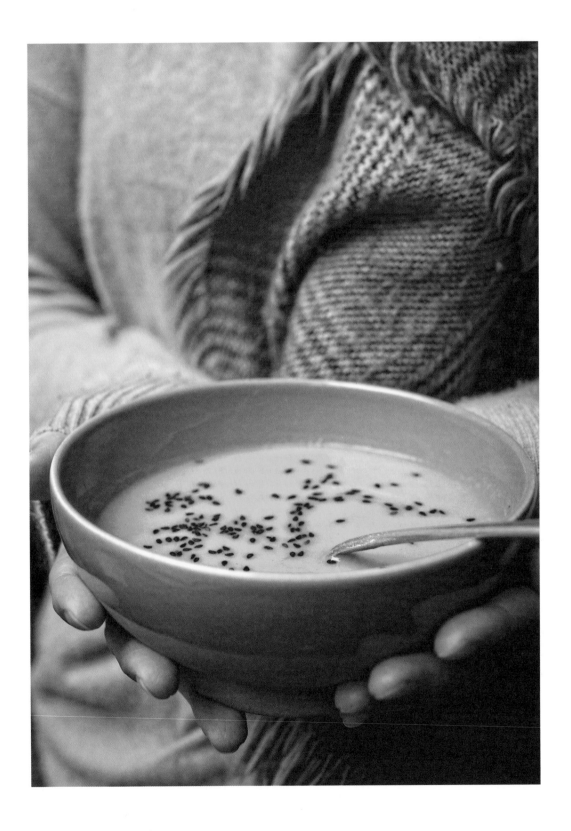

LEMONGRASS, COCONUT, AND SWEET POTATO SOUP

===

Lemongrass is the easiest of exotic Asian herbs to deal with in a Western kitchen. I tend to have problems pronouncing the others, let alone soliciting them into a pan. Lemongrass is widely available in supermarkets now, which means we are becoming either more courageous behind the apron or more mournful of our carefree days backpacking around Thailand.

Organic coconut milk is best because otherwise the milk can be hijacked with all sorts of preservatives and stabilizers. If you think this is just claptrap, I urge you to buy both and compare. You'll notice a trippy purple hue in many nonorganic milks.

Gently warm a dollop of extra virgin coconut oil in a sauté pan. Add the sweet potatoes, onions, and garlic and leave to sweat quietly while you prepare the remaining ingredients. This process sweetens the veggies naturally as long as you don't brown them.

Bash the fat, fibrous end of the lemongrass stalks with the base of a saucepan or other heavy object. Of course, a pestle and mortar would be perfect, but not as cathartic as a flying saucepan after a long day in the office. Add the smashed stalks to the sweet potatoes and onions along with the stock and coconut milk. Bring to a simmer and cook for 10 minutes, until soft.

Remove the lemongrass and discard. Purée the soup with a hand-held blender until delectably smooth. Tickle with cayenne to give delicious heat and a splash of lime for a sharp kick. Finally, dazzle with the torn cilantro, a splash of tamari, and your vacation photo album. Guaranteed to transport you straight back to the coconut-lined beaches of Koh Samui.

Good blob of extra virgin coconut oil
2 sweet potatoes, peeled and diced
1 onion, diced
3 garlic cloves, chopped
1-2 lemongrass stalks
2 cups (500 ml) vegetable stock or water
1 (400 g) can organic coconut milk
Pinch of cayenne (optional)
Squeeze of lime juice
Handful of fresh cilantro leaves, torn
Tamari, to serve

Serves 4

HITCHCOCK AND NUTMEG SOUP

================================

Thank goodness you can now buy raw pumpkin from supermarkets in wedges, just like melon. Hacking into a whole one is a little too Hitchcock for me. Besides, you'd need to be Mr. Universe to dice up a pumpkin.

Roasted, this saffron-colored vegetable is deliciously sweet and mapley to taste. As soon as you socialize it with your palate, you'll wonder why we eat it only at Halloween. Be careful not to buy the monstrous decorative pumpkins, which are good only for ghoulish faces.

Nuts like me-short for nutritionists-love pumpkin because of its supersonic carotenoids, its liver-loving antioxidants, and its astral amounts of vitamins C and A. Winter bugs won't stand a chance. Of particular importance to the hypertension-istas or balding men among us, pumpkin sports more potassium than the humble banana: five times as much.

2 onions, chopped
5 garlic cloves, left in their
  paper houses
1 pumpkin (2- to 3-lb)
Good splash of extra virgin
  olive or coconut oil
3-4 cups (up to 1 liter)
  chicken or vegetable stock
Whole nutmeg, to garnish
Buckwheat blini (page 48) to
  serve

Serves 8

Preheat the oven to 400°F (200°C).

Toss the chopped onions onto a large baking tray with the whole cloves of garlic in their papery pods. Slice the pumpkin into wedges, discard its stringy nest and seeds, and dice the flesh into bite-size pieces. Leave the skin on if it's an organic pumpkin. Tumble with the onions and garlic, giving it all a good lick of oil. (You may need to use 2 trays to avoid overcrowding.) Roast for 45 minutes, or until the pumpkin is soft and caramelized around the edges. Shake the tray once or twice during roasting, just so your nostrils can party.

Once the pumpkin is seriously tender and sweet, scoop into your food processor alongside your onions. You'll need to squeeze the garlic from their papery shells-swipe a little taste for yourself. It's pretty cosmic roasted this way. Blend on high. Add enough stock to achieve the desired consistency of your soup. Whiz carefully now, trying not to scald yourself or redec-orate the kitchen walls. Pour into big bowls and grate fresh nutmeg on top.

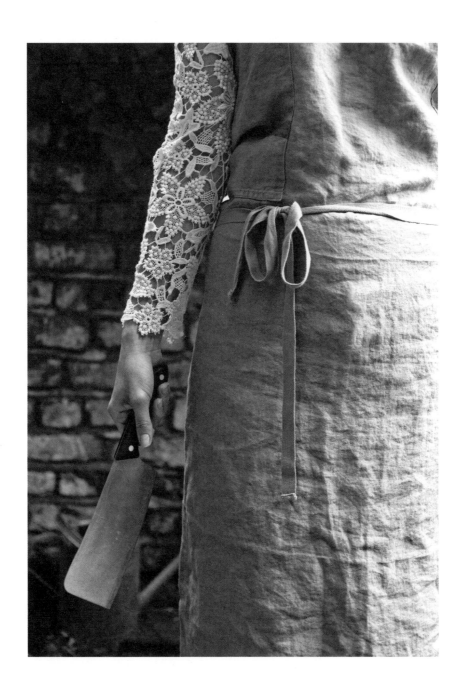

ROASTED GARLIC AND WILD NETTLE SOUP

===

Children are fascinated with nettle soup because it curiously fails to sting their tongue. Use this alleged sorcery to your advantage. If the kiddos stay up later than bedtime, threaten to turn them into purple ferrets. In the meantime, learn this recipe by heart so that when you return from the fields, the ingenious alchemy can begin.

1 whole head of garlic,
  cloves peeled
Glug of extra virgin olive oil
Sea salt flakes
Crack of black pepper
4 onions, diced
1 leek, chopped any old way
Roughly $^1/_2$ bag of nettle
  leaves*
8.5 cups (2 liters) homemade
  chicken or vegetable stock
1 cup (140 g) frozen peas
  (optional)

Serves 12

** Please use rubber gloves
when you pick the nettles!*

To roast the garlic, preheat your oven to 350°F (180°C).

Toss the garlic cloves in a bowl with the olive oil and seasoning. Stack 6 pieces of aluminum foil on a work surface and place a sheet of parchment paper on top. This prevents the garlic from coloring or burning and turning bitter. Put the cloves in the middle of the paper and fold the parchment and foil over it like a tent, scrunching the edges. Make sure it's sealed well. Place the package in the center of the oven and roast for 45 minutes.

Remove from the oven and allow to cool for at least 30 minutes. If you open the package too early, you will lose all that fabulous juice or burn yourself with plumes of steam.

If this all seems a little much, feel free to use crushed raw garlic in place of creamy roasted garlic. They taste very different but are both fabulous in their own ways.

To make the nettle soup, sweat the onions and leek in olive oil over gentle heat for 10 minutes, until the onions look translucent. If the veggies catch on the bottom of the pan and start burning, splash some water in and turn the heat down. Using a heavy-based saucepan is best.

Rinse the nettles under running water and remember to wear your rubber gloves. Spring nettles are sweetest. Toss the nettles into your pot of veggies and add the stock, salt flakes, and cracked pepper. Bring to a boil, immediately reduce the heat to a gurgling simmer, and cook for 5-6 minutes. Any longer, and you risk murdering the taste. Remove from the heat and sprinkle in the peas (if using). So sweet and juicy when fresh, baby peas

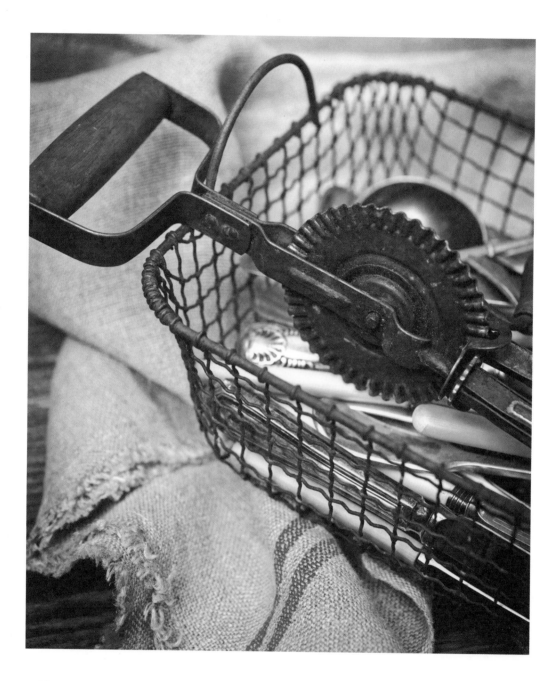

will cook rapidly in the residual heat of the soup. Take
out your immersion blender and whiz everything until
delectably smooth. Mash the roasted garlic and stir it
through. This soup also freezes well and sings beside a
slice of toasted rye sourdough.

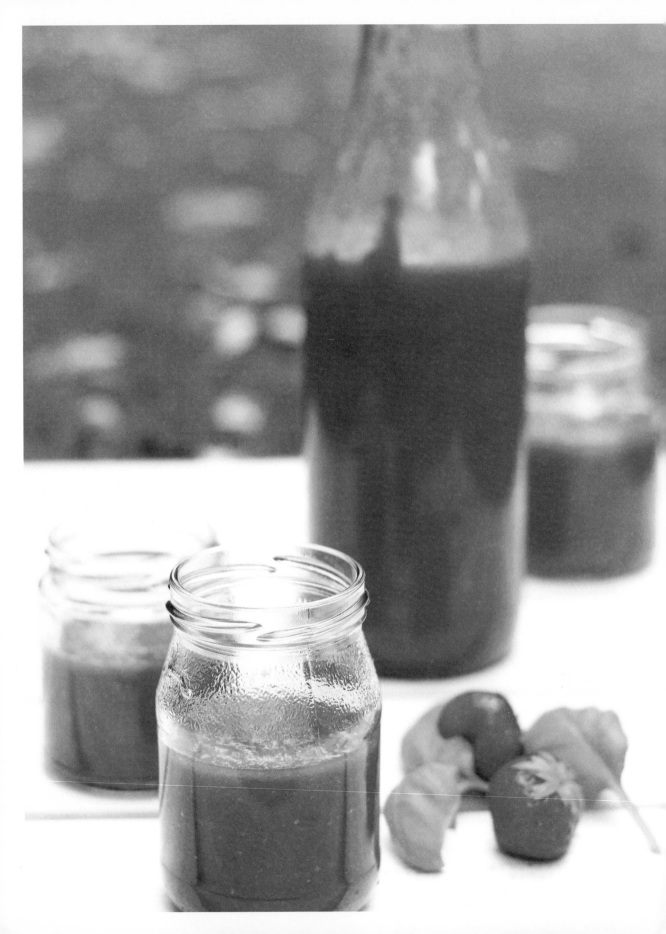

PICNIC GAZPACHO

==================

Tomatoes practically blush with virtue, like a rosy cherub with puppy fat. You've probably noticed the praise they enjoy in medical circles. In fact, the European Commission is backing a five-year research project called Lycocard to explore the role that tomatoes play in reducing the risk of developing cardiovascular disease and prostate cancer.

Lycopene, a carotenoid found in tomatoes, is thought to have raging antioxidant properties. We like antioxidants because they help counteract mischief-making oxidants in our bloodstream. These meddlesome oxidants are often the result of poor dietary choices like processed fats, sugar, artificial additives, and synthetically created preservatives. Cheap pre-packaged meals are full of the above, making your blood feel like sludge.

Now that we know lycopene can help zap villainous oxidants, we should be plotting to take more. Gazpacho is a chilled tomato soup. It's absurdly refreshing on a summer's day, especially if heat tends to muffle your appetite. When temperatures soar, the Spanish swill pitchers of gazpacho. Their tickers are all the merrier for it.

Too simple, really-whiz and serve. You'll need to start with the cherry tomatoes and garlic. Just give them a jolly good whiz in a high-speed blender until they're really smooth. Add in the spring onions, red pepper, cucumber, passata, lemon juice, and a crack of black pepper and pulse very briefly. Gazpacho is best when it's thick and chunky, like a soupy salsa. If you accidently purée until kingdom come, don't panic. Blame heat stroke. Garnish with a smile and crumbled egg, announcing that it is in fact salmorejo.

Chill in the refrigerator for at least 1 hour and spoon into 4 shallow soup bowls. Serve with a drizzle of top-quality olive oil, ice cubes, a few basil leaves and The Gypsy Kings' greatest hits.

1 pint (250 g) cherry
  tomatoes, quartered
2 garlic cloves, crushed
3 spring onions, sliced
1 red bell pepper, deseeded
  and diced
1 cup diced cucumber
2 cups tomato passata or
  crushed tomatoes
Juice of 1 small lemon
Fresh crack of black pepper
Top-quality extra virgin
  olive oil, to serve
Ice cubes, to serve
Basil leaves, to garnish
  (optional)

Serves 4

SMOKY BLACK BEAN SOUP

===============================

I love this soup. Your taste buds will backflip and your cardiologist is sure to wildly applaud. We already know the virtues of beans. Add to this tomatoes' heart-protective carotenoids, olive oil's cholesterol-busting tendencies, and yeast flakes' cargo of B vitamins, and you've got yourself a defibrillator in a kitchen pot. Just don't leave out the cumin or smoked paprika. They give this soup an extraterrestrial kick.

2-3 cups (200-300 g) chopped
  leeks
1 garlic clove, sliced (not
  crushed)
4 tablespoons extra virgin
  olive oil
1 teaspoon ground cumin
1 teaspoon smoked paprika
Two 15 oz(400 g) cans black
  beans, drained and rinsed
One 14 oz (400 g) can of
  cherry tomatoes
6 cups (1.5 liters) vegetable
  stock or seasoned water
1 tablespoon tomato purée
1 tablespoon nutritional
  yeast flakes (optional)
1-2 teaspoons honey or
  coconut sugar
Splash of tamari

For the pseudo crème fraîche:
1 cup (250 ml) natural or
  coconut yogurt
1 garlic clove, crushed
Handful of parsley, chopped
A few turns of the black
  pepper mill

Serves 6-8

Using a large heavy-based saucepan on low heat, sweat the leeks, garlic, and olive oil for 8-10 minutes, until soft and sweet. Toss in your cumin and smoked paprika and stir briskly, allowing their aroma to hit your hungry nostrils, then add the remaining ingredients. Turn the heat up until the soup starts to gurgle, cover, and lower the heat again. Allow to putter away for 5 minutes.

Ladle into large bowls and top with a pseudo "crème fraîche" made from natural yogurt, crushed garlic, parsley, and smashed black pepper.

CHILLED AVOCADO AND WATERCRESS SOUP

===

Instead of artery-clogging cream, you'll find that avocado can deliciously thicken soup while cranking up your meal's nutritional value. Avocados are especially high in vitamin E, nature's antidote to damaged skin. Combined with this soup's stellar vitamin C content, you're looking at an antiaging elixir. Although I'm not suggesting you apply it as a face mask.

Many of us need to increase our calcium intake from sources other than dairy. Watercress should help.

Start by gently warming the olive oil in a large pan. Add your onion and garlic to the oil and cook on low for around 10 minutes, until the onion looks fairly translucent. This process is called sweating and helps to sweeten root vegetables for soups.

Add the peas, watercress, and stock. Cook for 5 minutes, until the water starts to violently boil. Remove from the heat and pulse with a hand-held blender. It will turn a brilliant green. Pour into a wide-brimmed, pre-chilled bowl and allow to cool in the fridge for 1 hour. An ice bath is helpful.

Preheat the oven to 350°F (180°C). Toast the almonds on a flat oven tray for 4–6 minutes, until lightly colored but not brown. Set aside.

Once the soup is chilled, scoop out the flesh of your chilled avocado and add before serving. Give everything another blitz and serve immediately with an untidy smattering of toasted almonds.

2 tablespoons extra virgin olive oil
1 onion, diced
2 garlic cloves, minced
4 cups (450 g) frozen peas
1 regular bunch (125 g) watercress
4 cups (1 liter) homemade vegetable or chicken stock
Flaked almonds, to serve (optional)
1 medium avocado, chilled

Serves 4

90-SECOND BARLEY MISO SOUP

====================================

Miso is one of Japan's culinary trophies. Made from fermenting soy beans or grains with a live culture, miso is high in enzymes, good bacteria, female-friendly isofla-vones, cancer-fighting selenium, and that elusive vitamin B12. Look for unpas-teurized miso in the refrigerated section of all good food stores. You'll notice there are lots of varieties and grains to choose from, a bit like wine. Some are sweet, others are earthy and full bodied. I've even noticed happy versions with fermented hemp for the die-hard hippies among us.

Miso paste is my secret weapon in the kitchen. When a sauce, soup, or dressing misbehaves, in goes a tablespoon of barley miso and out comes Beethoven's seventh symphony.

A small nutritional caveat-never boil fresh miso. Its flavor and bacterial culture will get the guillotine. Instead, add a little of the liquid to a cup with the miso and dissolve into a smooth paste. Pour this brew back into the soup or sauce and then serve without any further cooking.

1-2 teaspoons unpasteurized
  barley (or other) miso
1 spring onion, sliced
Sprinkle of peas
1 quail's egg (optional)
Pinch of arame seaweed
  (soaked for 10 minutes) or
  nori flakes

Serves 1

Mix the miso paste in a soup bowl with 2 tablespoons of hot water until dissolved. Pour over boiled water from the kettle and add the spring onions and peas. Crack a raw quail's egg into the center (if using). The heat from the soup will quickly cook the teeny tiny egg. It's pretty awesome to watch.

If that doesn't appeal, play with additions such as warm almond milk, soaked arame, or nori flakes. Reach into the freezer and grab a slice of Your New Wheat-Free Bread (page 51). No need to cook tonight.

JEWISH PENICILLIN

========================

There's nothing quite like a bubbling cauldron of chicken stock wafting through the kitchen on a cold winter evening. Sends my nostrils into a frenzy of hunger. Stock is quite happy to sit on the stovetop and gurgle away for several hours, enveloping your senses while you get going on that box set of The Wire.

Let's be honest: most of us still grab ready-made stock cubes instead of making our own. But that's like comparing Justin Bieber to Eric Clapton. The first ingredient in an average chicken stock cube is salt. What a rip-off. Then comes artery-clogging hydrogenated fat, followed by sugar-exclamation mark-unspecified starch (aka more sugar), monosodium glutamate (MSG), and dubious "flavorings." Even the canned varieties are based on these cheap, phony stocks.

This recipe is liquid gold. Simmering the bones helps draw out the chicken's natural minerals and collagen to fuel our bodies. Its potency is further enhanced with garlic, ginger, and turmeric's antiviral, antibacterial, and anti-inflammatory compounds. Our grannies and our granny's grannies used it to soothe indolent limbs and hazy eyes in place of popping flu pills.

Ask your local butcher to save his free-range or organic chicken carcasses for you instead of dumping them. Just make sure to return his generosity with a great big flask of steaming hot goodness and a seraphic smile.

Break up your chicken carcass as much as you can and cover with cold filtered water in a large saucepan. Add all the ingredients to the pot and bring to a "shy" simmer, uncovered. Lower the heat so that the liquid is only shuddering. Skim off and discard the foam that appears on the surface over the next 60 minutes—there's no need to become a slave to it, however.

Once the broth has a rich, chickeny flavor, usually in 4-24 hours, turn off the heat. Strain. Allow the broth to settle and throw out the bones and veggies. Store in the freezer to make soup at a later date or dive straight in.

Give this stock your own signature stamp by adding grilled mushrooms, slices of avocado and chili, broken buckwheat noodles, or freshly chopped parsley before serving. Although it's so darn delicious on its own, it rarely needs any doctoring.

1 organic chicken carcass

3 onions, peeled and roughly chopped

3 celery sticks, roughly chopped

5 garlic cloves, peeled

2 bay leaves

Thumb-sized piece of fresh ginger, peeled and chopped

1-inch piece of fresh turmeric root, peeled

1 teaspoon unrefined salt flakes

Freshly cracked black pepper, to serve

3 tablespoons apple cider vinegar

Makes 1-2 liters

Salads

Healthy eating should never tax your taste buds.

Relax. You're in the right place. Cleaning up your diet doesn't
need to involve neon leotards or cauliflower smoothies.
No one should be threatened with that. This chapter is more
about pleasure than denial. We could all improve
our diets, but we don't have to sacrifice flavor.

The food we eat is inescapably linked to our concentration levels,
our mood, our libido, and yes, our love handles.
We eat about five times a day. That's over 1,800 opportunities
each year to positively affect our energy and weight.
Salads are a great place to start. Let me prove it.

SPIRALIZER RECIPES - MAKING SPAGHETTI FROM ZUCCHINI

ooooooooooooooooooooooooooooooooooooooooooooooooooooooooo

I love spiralizers. These dinky machines make you feel like David Copperfield in the kitchen. Instead of prepping pasta, you can grab a zucchini, fix it to a spiralizer, and *kaboom*! Zucchini spaghetti! And if you don't fancy forking out for another kitchen gadget, you could use a potato peeler to scrape ribbons from the vegetables instead.

A naturally shy vegetable, zucchini carry flavor rather than provide it. The trick is to avoid the large, bitter ones. You can dress zucchini spaghetti up with your usual crushed tomatoes, a bit of garlic, olives, spinach, and look! That's your five-a-day busted in less time than it takes to reheat a dodgy take-out. Investing in a spiralizer might be the best twenty-five dollars you'll spend this year.

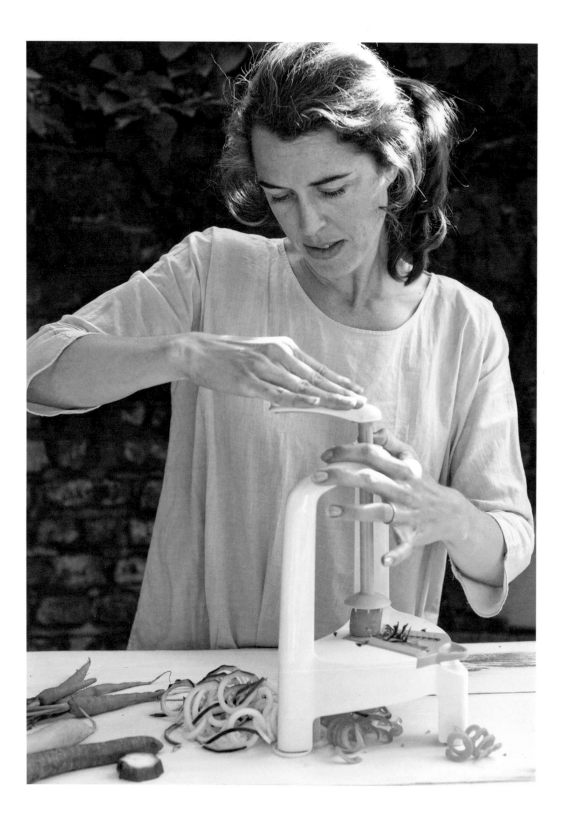

SPIRALIZER RECIPES - THE HAPPY ZUCCHINI

OOOOOOOOOOOOOOOOOOOOOOOOOOOOOOOOOOOOOOOOOOOOOOO

Crunchy, smooth, and zippy, this is one happy zucchini.

1 fat carrot
1 small to medium zucchini
$^1/_4$ cup (4 tablespoons)
  walnuts
$^1/_4$ cup (4 tablespoons) dried
  cranberries
Handful of flat-leaf parsley,
  dill, or chervil

For the dressing:
3 tablespoons organic natural
  soy yogurt
2 tablespoons red wine
  vinegar or apple cider
  vinegar
1 tablespoon Dijon mustard
$^1/_2$ garlic clove, minced

Serves 2 as a main or 3 as a
  side

Spiralize the carrot and zucchini into a large bowl.
Loosely toss together with the walnuts, cranberries
(raisins and grapes love this recipe too), and herbs.

To make the dressing, whisk together the yogurt,
vinegar, mustard, and garlic. Tumble into the prepared
carrot and zucchini. Dig in.

SPIRALIZER RECIPES - WASABI PEA CARBONARA

○○

This is a good creamy dish with a delicious sting of wasabi. When you're rehydrating dried mango, just add enough water for them to soak it up. Leave for a few hours, or overnight if possible.

Pour boiling hot water on top of the frozen peas and leave to sit while you spiralize the zucchini and carrot into a bowl. Drain and add the peas to your zucchini and carrot spaghetti.

In a separate bowl, purée the avocado, the rehydrated mango pieces and their soaking liquid, the wasabi, green tea (if using), and the lemon or lime juice. Taste, and add a dash more juice if you think it's required. Pour this sumptuous green ganache over the zucchini spaghetti and coat it thoroughly. If you think there is too much sauce, spiralize another carrot into the mix.

Divide between bowls and have your friends guess the ingredients!

$^1/_2$ cup (70 g) frozen peas
1 small to medium zucchini
1 fat carrot
Flesh of 1 avocado
Handful of dried mango,
  rehydrated in water
  (see note above)
2 teaspoons organic wasabi
  paste
1 teaspoon matcha green tea
  powder (optional)
Squeeze of lemon or lime juice

Serves 4-5 as a starter or
  side

SPIRALIZER RECIPES - FLAKED SALMON WITH SPICY POMEGRANATE NOODLES

○○

One of my all-time favorite salads. The key lies in good-quality pomegranate molasses, so beware of imposters!

2 fillets organic salmon or
   wild trout
Extra virgin raw coconut oil
   (or whatever oil you prefer)
1 fat carrot
1 small to medium zucchini
2 tablespoons pomegranate
   molasses
2 tablespoons almond butter
2 tablespoons cold-pressed
   toasted sesame oil
2 tablespoons Bragg Liquid
   Aminos or 1 tablespoon
   tamari
1 small garlic clove, minced
   or crushed
Good pinch of cayenne pepper
Pomegranate seeds, to garnish

Serves 2

Preheat the oven to 400°F (200°C).

Prepare the salmon by wrapping the fillets in a parcel of aluminum foil and drizzle with the oil. I use extra virgin raw coconut oil, but use whatever you're happiest with. Make sure there's lots of space above the fillets- it's more like a tent than a parcel. They steam in their own juices this way.

Transfer the tent of salmon onto a baking tray and roast for 10-15 minutes, depending on how big the fillets are. Check by pulling the flesh apart. If they're not done, just reseal your tent and pop them in the oven again. When you've become familiar with this method of cooking, crank it up another level by adding smashed lemon-grass, maple syrup, chili, cumin, kaffir lime leaves, or whatever tickles your appetite on any given evening.

While the salmon is cooking, spiralize the carrot and zucchini. In a separate bowl, beat together the remaining ingredients to make your spicy dressing. Toss through your spiralized noodles and divide between 2 bowls. When the salmon is done to your liking, flake the flesh over each bowl of noodles, then sprinkle over the pomegranate seeds. Awesome meal on a warm summer evening.

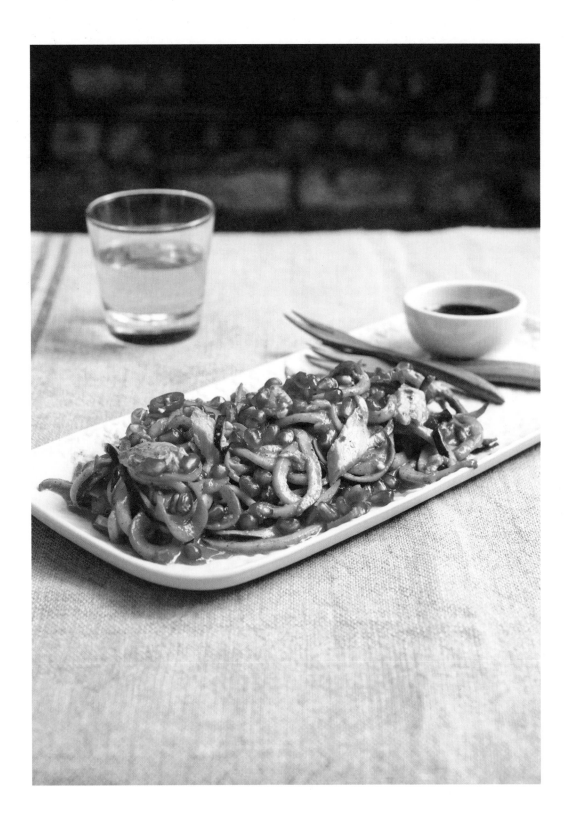

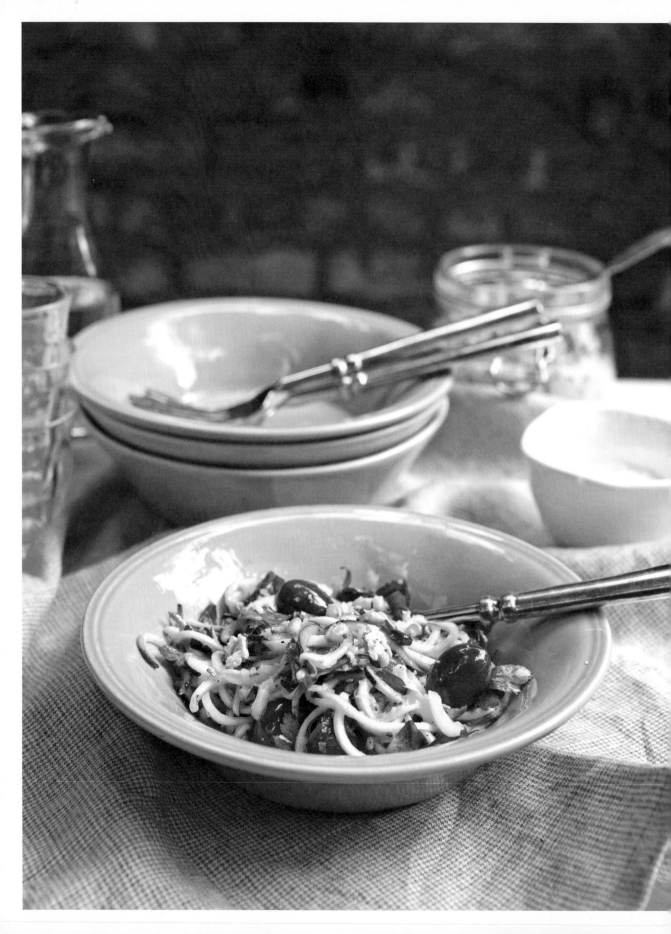

SPIRALIZER RECIPES - GARLICKY TAGLIATELLE WITH BLACK OLIVES AND PINE NUT RICOTTA

○○○

Sick of stodgy pasta and cheese? Preparing zucchini and carrot tagliatelle takes less time than boiling pasta, and also delivers your entire vegetable RDA. Admittedly the pine nut ricotta demands a bit of Mary Poppins in the kitchen, but if you plug in some Ricky Martin he'll visit your fingertips. My hubby sneaks some diced anchovies and tomatoes in here too.

Put the zucchini and carrot through the middle blade of your spiralizer or use a potato peeler to create long, thin ribbons.

In a separate bowl, whisk together the parsley, garlic, olive oil, and lemon juice. You won't need it all, so freeze the remainder for another evening.

Tumble enough of the dressing into your tagliatelle and toss thoroughly to coat each strand. Sprinkle in the chopped olives. Crown with a generous drop of pine nut ricotta and a few turns of the black pepper mill.
A simple smattering of pumpkin seeds is a filling alternative to the ricotta.

1 zucchini
1 carrot
Roughly $1/2$ cup flat-leaf parsley or chervil
3 garlic cloves, crushed or finely grated
$1/2$ cup (125 ml) extra virgin olive oil
Juice and zest of 2 small lemons
Handful of black olives, roughly chopped
Pine nut ricotta (page 143) or pumpkin seeds

Serves 2

SPIRALIZER RECIPES - RED PEPPER AND WALNUT (MUHAMMARA) NOODLES

ooooooooooooooooooooooooooooooooooooooooooooooooooooooooooooooooo

Last time I made these noodles, I necked the entire batch. My husband's roar was heard several postcodes away.

2 fat carrots
2 small to medium zucchini
3 red peppers (or 1 jar of
  roasted peppers)
1 cup (120 g) walnuts
$^1/_3$ cup (25 g) preferred
  breadcrumbs
3 garlic cloves, minced and
  mashed to a paste with $^1/_2$
  teaspoon salt flakes
4 tablespoons tomato purée
1 tablespoon pomegranate
  molasses
1 teaspoon ground cumin
pinch of dried chili flakes
$^1/_2$ cup extra virgin olive oil
Fresh lemon juice, to taste
  (optional)

Serves 6 as a starter or side

Spiralize the carrots and zucchini. Large zucchini can taste bitter and fluffy, so it's worth hunting down the smaller ones.

Let's get making the muhammara. To prep the peppers, place them directly on the middle shelf in a very hot oven. Let them roast for around 40 minutes, until they're on the brink of collapse. Don't worry if their skin is blistered or black. It's what's inside that counts. Gently remove the roasted peppers from the oven by pulling the stalk of each one and catching them in a large bowl. Cover the bowl with cling wrap for 10 minutes. This makes it much easier to remove their skins. Without ouching yourself, pinch off the skin and discard along with the stalks and seeds.

To prep the walnuts, smash them in a mortar with a pestle until their natural oils begin to be released. Or you could use the base of a saucepan, so long as the neighbors aren't in.

Purée the rest of the ingredients except the olive oil and lemon juice into a smooth, creamy dip. Now stir through the olive oil and then the walnuts.

Taste, and adjust with a squeeze of lemon or more chili flakes if you fancy. Tumble into your prepped noodles and divide between your serving bowls. Black olives and hummus make for groovy companions.

SPIRALIZER RECIPES - CURLY CARROTS

○○○

My boys chase each other with giant shoelaces of raw carrot. They think it's hilarious. I look on with the wonder of an astronomer sighting a new galaxy. Who would have thought raw carrots could be so much fun?

When they have playdates, Benjamin and Marty beg me to make "curly carrots" for their unsuspecting guests. Everyone ditches the Lego, sits on the floor and chomps on ribbons of carrots as if they were licorice laces.

Use the smallest plate on your spiralizer to make carrot laces. The carrot needs to be fat, or else you'll be left with brief curls of carrots instead of long, curly laces.

1 fat carrot
Some currants or pomegranate
  seeds

Makes 3-4 snack portions

SPIRALIZER RECIPES - CARROT RIBBONS AND SPRING PESTO

○○○

Leftover pesto can be frozen in jars. Make sure to press the pesto down firmly with the back of a spoon to remove any pockets of air (trapped air can cause contamination and foul tempers). Top the pesto with a little more oil, making a seal.

Start by picking over the wild garlic leaves and discarding any coarse stalks and grass. Whiz in a food processor along with the pumpkin seeds, olive oil, salt, and lemon juice. Transfer to a scrupulously clean jar and set aside. This takes 6 minutes, tops.

Head and tail the carrots. Make sure they are straight to facilitate smooth spiralizing. Put them through your spiralizer and collect the curly carrots in a bowl. Toss through the wild garlic pesto and dig in. It's honkingly good stuff. Use the smallest plate on your spiralizer to make carrot laces. The carrot needs to be fat, or else you'll be left with brief curls of carrots instead of long curly laces.

1 large bunch (50 g) freshly
  picked wild garlic leaves
3 tablespoons (25 g) pumpkin
  seeds
$^1/_2$ cup (125 ml) extra virgin
  olive oil
$^1/_2$ teaspoon sea salt flakes
Small squeeze of lemon or lime
  juice
2 fat carrots

Serves 2

MOON-DRIED TOMATOES AND SPROUTED HUMMUS

oooooooooooooooooooooooooooooooooooooooooooo

I'm a devotee of buying local and organic. This doesn't make me a sermonizing tree hugger or a hemp-wearing hippie (although I do have a crush on Woody Harrelson). I'm a fan because organic farming nourishes the soil naturally without the abuse of chemicals. Organic methods help protect Mother Nature's playground and preserve her biodiversity. (Though science is rarely ever that simple.)

By now you've probably heard about colony collapse disorder and the disappearance of honeybees in many parts of France, Britain, and the United States. This phenomenon has been increasingly linked to neonicotinoid insecticides. Not good news. Honeybees are critical for the pollination of many of our favorite foods, such as almonds, apples, beetroot, asparagus, and blueberries. Scientists say the disruption of pollination could wipe out entire crops, threaten our agriculture, and bring the world into an ecological crisis. According to the USDA, one-third of the American diet relies on bee pollination.

So what can we do? For a start, we can choose to support farmers who grow vegetables without the indiscriminate use of agrichemicals. Check out local organic farmers' markets. By doing so, we not only support our winged friends, we also support nature, our local economy, our health, and even our taste buds. Second, think about becoming a beekeeper. (The first might be easier to manage.) For more information, visit the beautiful site www.helpsavebees.co.uk.

For the moon-dried tomatoes:
About 16 cherry tomatoes,
  halved
1 garlic clove, finely chopped
3 tablespoons extra virgin
  olive oil
1 teaspoon coconut blossom
  sugar or maple syrup
$^1/_2$ teaspoon sea salt flakes
Handful of fresh cilantro
  leaves

For the sprouted hummus:
1 cup (225 g) dried chickpeas
1-2 garlic cloves, crushed
$^1/_2$ cup (125 ml) chilled water
4-8 tablespoons lemon juice
4 tablespoons tahini or
  cashew butter
2-3 tablespoons ground cumin
2 tablespoons extra virgin
  olive oil

Preheat the oven to 425°F (220°C).

Coat the halved tomatoes generously with the garlic, oil, sugar, and salt. Sit the tomatoes cut side up in an ovenproof dish and pour the remaining juices over them. Pop in the oven and immediately turn off the heat. Leave overnight or for a day without opening the door.

For the sprouted hummus, simply sprout your dried chickpeas by soaking them in water overnight. Drain them the following morning and place the chickpeas on damp paper towels along the windowsill for the day. When you return from the office, you can canter straight into your kitchen and whiz up this hummus. Purée everything except the herbs in your food processor for 3 minutes. Add more ice water to help loosen it up if necessary.

Herbs are best chopped finely and stirred through the

(continued)

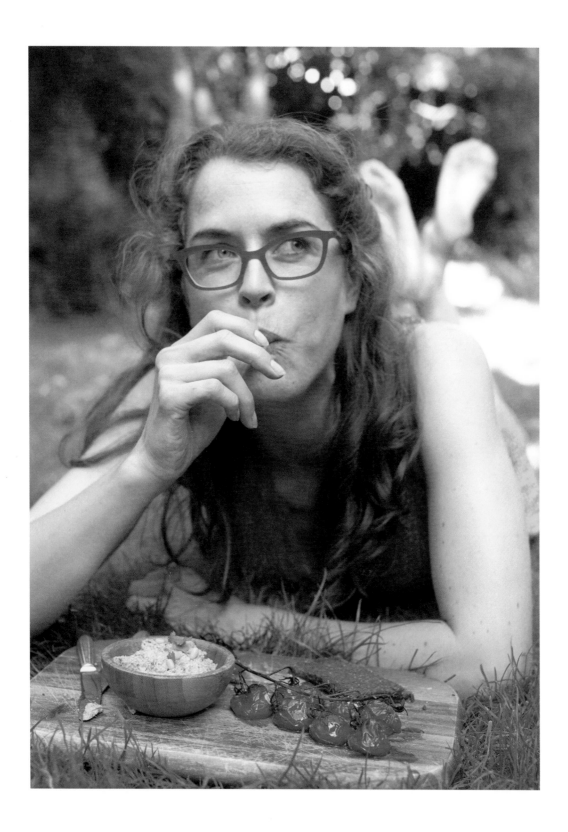

1 tablespoon tamari
$^1/_2$ cup finely chopped parsley,
   cilantro, basil, or black
   olives

Serves 4

hummus instead of blended. Otherwise, it can look as if Kermit the Frog crawled into your blender. The green tops of spring onions are a stealthy money-saver instead of using pricey fresh herbs.

Serve the tomatoes with loads of freshly chopped cilantro leaves and the sprouted hummus.

IRISH SUPERFOOD SALAD

○○○○○○○○○○○○○○○○○○○○○○○○○

This is a cosmic combo of truly tasty, local ingredients. It happens to be healthier and cheaper than popping vitamin pills. Plus you get to soak up the applause showered upon you by your dinner guests.

If you're feeling particularly lazy, use vacuum-packed beetroot in place of potatoes. No need for cooking.

Scrub and wash the baby potatoes, cover in cold salted water and bring to a boil for 15-20 minutes. Pierce them with a fork to check whether they are cooked. For the last 5 minutes of cooking the potatoes, add the eggs to cook simultaneously as a nifty time-saver. Once the eggs are boiled and the potatoes are cooked, drain and discard the cooking water. Allow to cool.

While the spuds are cooking, flake the mackerel fillet into a bowl with your chosen salad leaves, olive oil, the juice of half the lemon, lemon zest, nori flakes, and capers (if using).

Halve the cooked baby potatoes. Peel and quarter the boiled eggs. Gently toss everything together and serve straightaway or divide into paper deli boxes for lunch.

Handful of baby Irish
  potatoes
2 large eggs
1 fillet smoked mackerel
Handful of fresh arugula or
  watercress
Decent splash of extra virgin
  olive oil
Zest and juice of 1 small
  unwaxed lemon
Sprinkle of dried nori flakes
  (optional)
A few capers (optional)

Serves 3

BASIL BUTTER BEANS

oooooooooooooooooooo

We love butter beans because they look like something out of a Roald Dahl storybook. They're also cheap and keep in the cupboard for over a year. The trick with cooking beans is to soak them overnight. Unsoaked beans can taste dry and crunchy, even if you double the cooking time.

Here are a couple of tips to help you introduce butter beans to the dinner table: Toddlers will eat them whole. Teens don't notice them mixed through a can of baked beans. And leery grandparents won't suspect anything different in their mashed potatoes (FYI, butter beans mash beautifully). For everyone else, this recipe is sure to convert them.

1 cup (170 g) dried butter
  beans
3 tablespoons extra virgin
  olive oil
Zest of 1 small lemon
A few basil leaves, chopped

Serves 4 as a side

Cover the butter beans with water and soak overnight. The next day, drain the beans, cover with fresh unsalted water, and boil for 90 minutes, until very tender. Taste a bean-you're aiming for the texture of a baked potato. When you're satisfied, drain the beans and stir through the remaining ingredients. Also excellent with dribbly tomatoes and mint.

DINING AL DESKO BEET SALAD

OOOOOOOOOOOOOOOOOOOOOOOOOOOOO

I love the summer. It's probably my favorite day of the year. I queue up to sit in the park and sear my beautiful blue skin. For the other 364 days of the Irish calendar, I like to keep toasty indoors and dine al desko. Loads of us do it.

But keep those sandwiches away from me or I'll be snoring by 3 p.m. Food should give you energy, not take it away. Try this recipe and see for yourself. The ginger will give your circulation a good giddy up.

Chop the veggies into bite-size chunks. Two or three beets should suffice, depending on their size. Quantities are up to you.

Steam the chunks of carrot until tender. They won't need more than 5 minutes in a pot with a tightly covered lid and a minimum amount of water. You could also leave them raw for extra nutrition and crunch, but this renders talking over lunchtime next to impossible.

Toss the veggies, apple, and walnuts together with a splash of olive oil and a squeeze of lemon juice. Grate some ginger over everything using the same part of the grater that you would use for lemon zest. Taste, and adjust the seasoning to your liking. Wrestle into a plastic lunchbox or empty container. Just don't forget the fork.

2-3 cooked beets
1 large carrot
1 celery stalk
$1/2$ apple, diced
Handful of walnuts
Splash of olive oil
Squeeze of lemon juice
1-inch piece of fresh ginger, peeled
Salt and pepper

Serves 2

"F%*K ME" SALAD

ooooooooooooooo

*Here's a fragrant supper of fiery prawns, honeyed papaya, and mint, all kissed with toasted sesame oil. Anyone who tastes it usually responds with a whispered "f%*k me!"*

Chilis are devious little vegetables. They raise our body temperature and help release natural endorphins to keep our blood gurgling with excitement. I recommend the powdered form to give your lips a delicious sting and swell the senses. Guessing the heat of a fresh chili is riskier than cycling backward in a Grand Prix.

Rice or mung noodles for 2
1 small papaya
¹/₄ cucumber
¹/₄ red onion
12 cooked prawns
Freshly torn mint leaves

For the Thai dressing:
Juice of 1 lime
1 tablespoon fish sauce
 (nam pla)
1 tablespoon toasted
 sesame oil
2 teaspoons raw honey or
 maple syrup
Pinch of cayenne or
 freshly sliced chili

Serves 2

Cook the noodles according to the manufacturer's instructions on the packet (these can vary greatly). Cut the papaya in half, and again into slices. This will make it easier to cut into chunks for the salad. Treat it like a melon. While the seeds are deemed edible, they are deeply unpleasant. Known for its rich enzymes and potent anti-inflammatory compounds, papaya will help keep your liver on speaking terms with you. Especially if you're Irish.

Slice the cucumber thickly, then cut each slice into quarters. Slice the red onion thinly into rings. Toss the papaya, cucumber, and red onion joyfully together with the prawns and mint.

Whisk together the remaining ingredients to make a Thai dressing good enough to drink. Pour over your medley of papaya and allow the flavors to infuse. By now, your noodles will be ready. Drain and rinse briefly with cold water to separate the starchy bits. Tumble into the happy medley and serve with a fork and straw. If you're bringing this into work, expect office pillagers to descend. Arm yourself with an extra sharp fork.

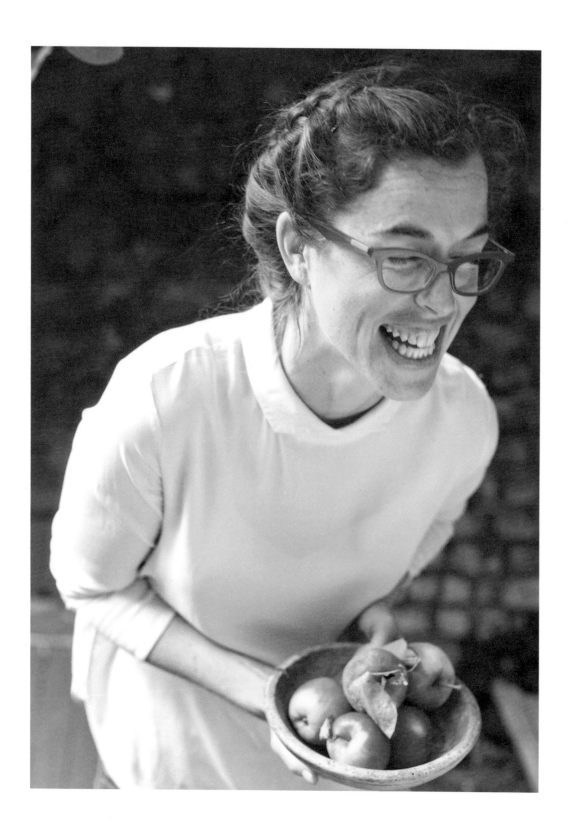

SAY HELLO TO OCEAN VEGGIES

ooooooooooooooooooooooooooooooooo

Seaweed is the next big thing. We Irish seem to think it's only useful for deflecting annoying children on the beach. In fact, seaweed is full of antiaging nutrients and disease-fighting lignans.

Listen up, rusty bones! Sea veggies' calcium supply is good for healthy bones and teeth, without the artery-clogging effects that dairy-rich diets can yield. Then there's iron—a mere 10 grams of mixed sea vegetables can give you just under half the recommended daily allowance of this blood-building mineral.

There are many types of sea vegetables to choose from, guaranteed to make the beach more exciting this year. Here are a few to get you started. All are harvested wild and are free from chemicals, preservatives, and, yes, sometimes taste.

The most common type of sea vegetable on our menus is <u>nori</u>, the shiny green wrapping around sushi. Nori is unusually rich in protein. You'll get loads of nori in Asian food stores for a fraction of the high street price. Best crumbled on top of brown rice.

<u>Agar</u> and <u>carrageen</u> are used in place of artificial stabilizers and gelling agents. I use them to set panna cotta and fruit jellies-a crafty way of getting important minerals into children's party food.

<u>Kombu</u> and <u>sugar kelp</u> are the dark ones that gave me nightmares as a nipper. Thick, slippery strands of goodness. Who would have thought? Pop them into slow-cooking stews at the very beginning. I find they can take a long time to break down. It's rumored that adding kombu to beans can help reduce incidences of trouser trumpets. That's Latin for flatulence.

I always add <u>wakame</u> to stews about 30 minutes before cooking is finished. It brings a good smack of umami for the taste buds as well as a suite of fancy minerals. Like most ocean veggies, a packet of wakame will last 3 years in the cupboard.

<u>Dulse</u> is particular to Ireland. This sea veggie has a chewy texture and deep purple hue. Best purchased in powdered form and sprinkled on food. The more courageous cooks can play with it in broths and soups.

<u>Arame</u> is the sweetest and most elegant of the sea vegetables. Jet-black angel strands of goodness. No need to cook-simply soak for 10 minutes and socialize them with broccoli, Brazil nuts, and soy sauce for a speedy lunch, or with sautéed garlic mushrooms as a side.

SESAME SEA SALAD

OOOOOOOOOOOOOOOOO

Arame doesn't taste as weird as it sounds. It is the easiest and prettiest seaweed to prepare. Consider it essential for your kitchen's emergency stash, specially designed for occasions when the oven decides to misbehave and you have a hot date to feed. Or a starving in-law. Equally as terrifying.

Handful (20 g) of dried arame
3 carrots, grated
3 spring onions, chopped
1/2 apple, grated
Juice of 1/2 lemon
3 tablespoons sesame seeds
3 tablespoons currants
3 tablespoons extra virgin
  olive or sesame oil

Serves 4 as a side dish

Soak the arame in cool filtered water for 10-15 minutes.

Meanwhile, toss together the grated carrots, spring onions, apple, lemon juice, sesame seeds, and currants. Gloss it up with a good splash of olive or sesame oil. When the sea veggie has swelled to twice its size, discard the water and comb through the salad. Serve alongside fish or hummus. Watch out, though-kids tend to spit out the spring onions!

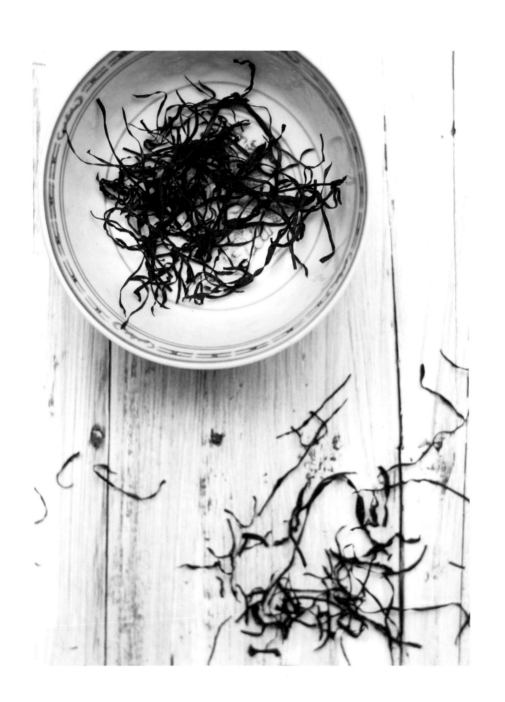

SPROUTING - THE BEAN ZOO

ooooooooooooooooooooooooooo

Here's a new hobby for a healthier, glossier you.

The task? (1) Purchase a three-tier germinator for about the same price as a yoga class. (2) Stock up on dried mung beans, alfalfa seeds, and whole lentils. These are the easiest chaps to start with. (3) In each tier, sprinkle 2 tablespoons of your chosen bean, seed, or lentil. (4) Let the germinator pay homage to the natural sunlight adorning your windowsill and tickle with water twice daily. Ta-da! Your very own bean zoo, providing oodles of entertainment, fascination, and nutrition.

Depending on the bean, seed, or lentil, sprouting can take from as little as 36 hours to 7 days. Your jolly germinator will come with an index of sprouting timelines. The trick is to refrigerate them as soon as they have sprouted, preventing them from growing too large and bitter. The shorter the sprouting time, the crunchier and sweeter they taste.

Bean sprouts provide a talented array of protein, vitamins, minerals, and raw enzymes without the hassle of cooking. This is what I call *real* fast food. Word of wisdom-don't bother trying egg, fish, or flaxseed oil with sprouts. Something alarmingly unpleasant happens.

SUPERMAN'S SALAD

ooooooooooooooooo

Choose from eight different varieties of sprouts to vivify your lunchtime and your liver. All sprouts need is a little lick of olive oil, juicy fruit, and chopped herbs before being thrown into Tupperware.

Take about 4 segments of grapefruit and peel the white pith away from the juicy flesh. Chop each segment into approximately 4 pieces. This could take a while—my grapefruit usually finds its way into my mouth. Roughly tear your chosen herbs and toss with the grapefruit, sprouts, and olive oil.

1 pink grapefruit
Handful of fresh chives,
   mint, or cilantro
1 mug of sprouted beans
2 tablespoons extra virgin
   olive oil

Serves 1-2

Further combos to try:
In place of pink grapefruit and chives, try olives, lemon juice, and parsley; chopped banana, coconut flakes, and cilantro; Brazil nuts, steamed broccoli and soy sauce; roasted veggies and arugula; yogurt, curry powder, raisins, and grated carrot; tofu, rice noodles, chili, and sesame oil; or avocado, pistachios, and dried apricots.

NECTARINE AND LITTLE GEM SALAD WITH GOJI BERRY CREAM

OOOOOOOOOOOOOOOOOOOOOOOOOOOOOOOOOOOOOOOOOOOOOOOOOOOOOOOOO

1-2 Little Gem lettuces
$1/2$ apple or nectarine,
   depending on the season
Handful of pumpkin seeds
Handful of sunflower seeds
A few turns of the black
   pepper mill

For the dressing:
6 tablespoons extra virgin
   olive oil
2 tablespoons lemon juice or
   apple cider vinegar
2 tablespoons goji berries
1 tablespoon raw honey, brown
   rice syrup, or raw agave
   nectar
Pinch of cayenne

Serves 2

Break the leaves from the lettuce heads into the largest bowl you have. Gently tumble with the chopped apple, seeds, and black pepper. You can toast the seeds to bring out their nuttiness: heat a nonstick pan on high and toast the seeds for 30 seconds. They are done when you hear the pumpkin seeds pop off the pan. A few chili flakes will give a delicious nip.

Using a hand-held blender, purée the dressing ingredients to make a glossy sauce almost like a mayo but lighter in consistency. If your blender is as contrary as mine, it's worth soaking the goji berries in a little water first for 25 minutes. This should make the ride a little smoother. Pour over the salad and lightly toss together using your fingertips. An implement like a spoon or a fork can bruise the leaves and make a salad quickly look tired.

Pile on the center of a large plate. A turn or two of the black pepper mill is all it needs now. And maybe a bit of adulation. The pine nut ricotta on page 143 is fairly swell on top.

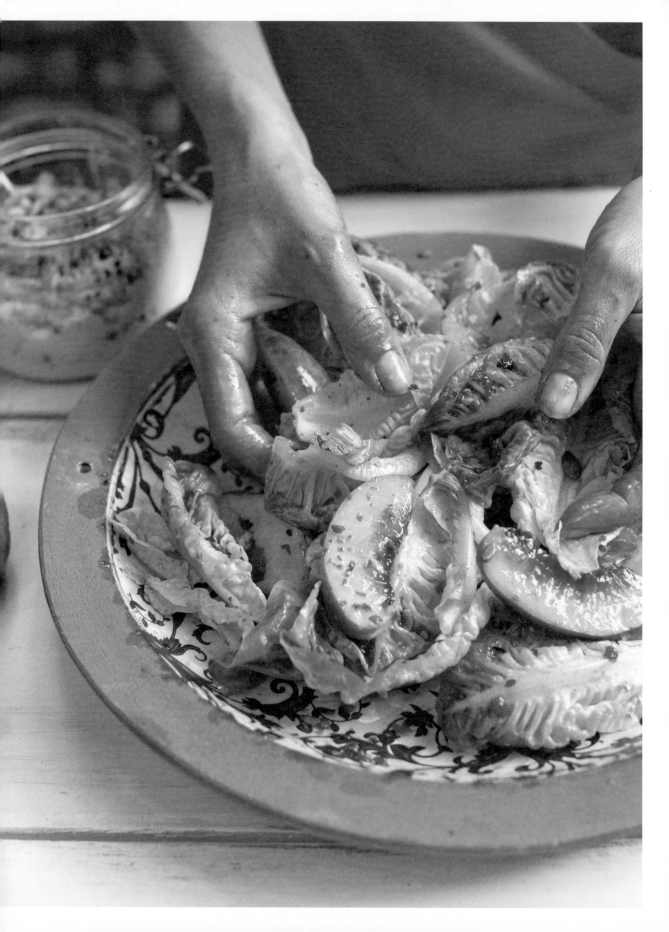

BOND GIRL SALAD

oooooooooooooooooo

If we are what we eat, then most people are cheap, fast, and easy. But good nutrition doesn't have to compromise your wallet or your wristwatch. Raging hot actress Halle Berry swears by her five-factor rule: meals have to use five different ingredients and be ready to eat in five minutes.

A few examples: smoked salmon, poached egg, fresh cress, cucumber, and jarred capers; grated raw carrot, coconut, sultanas, curry powder, and sesame oil; or canned mackerel, spring onion, arugula, tomato, and avocado. Your brain gets a good workout! No refined muck, of course, just five wholesome ingredients. That means if you couldn't find a particular ingredient one hundred years ago, it doesn't count.

Try this Indonesian-style slaw to get you started. It takes a lot less than five minutes to make and is a great side dish with fish.

3 handfuls of finely sliced
  red cabbage
1 cup (150 g) chopped
  pineapple
$^1/_2$ cup (125 ml) natural yogurt
$^1/_4$ cup (35 g) sultanas
1 tablespoon curry powder
Sprinkling of red-skinned
  peanuts

Serves 2-3

Tumble all the ingredients together. If you have a red onion loitering in the pantry, throw that in too. Use whatever natural yogurt you have—coconut, soy, goat, sheep. The hotter the curry powder is, the better. Something cosmic happens to pineapple when fire touches its orbit.

PROBIOTIC CELERIAC SLAW

oooooooooooooooooooooooooooo

Celeriac may look like a Harry Potter concoction, but it's actually as common as turnips. Watch out for it on your next trip to the grocer's. You'll notice that the rest of these ingredients are probably resident in your fridge already, save the offensive-sounding berry. Physalis look like massive amber raisins and have a sherbety smack.

Sprightly little berries buzzing with goodness and charm, physalis supply immune-enhancing beta-carotene and vitamin C to help slay bugs. Throw them into salads and conversation to impress. However, it would be prudent to enunciate carefully. Get it wrong, and you will sound as if you enjoy STDs.

If you want to upgrade the quantities of this slaw for a party, the ratio of apple to carrot to celeriac is 3:2:1. In other words, remember to grate three times the amount of apple to the amount of grated celeriac. You're in control.

Let all the ingredients converse in a large bowl. If you're planning on having leftovers the next day, dunk more yogurt into the slaw before plating up. There's no need for additional probiotic powder-you'll get plenty in the natural yogurt. I originally devised this recipe for a client finishing several courses of antibiotics, so we whacked up the probiotic element to nourish her intestinal flora.

$^3/_4$ cup (65 g) grated apple
$^1/_2$ cup (40 g) grated carrot
$^1/_2$ cup (80 g) whole walnuts, finely chopped
$^1/_2$ cup (125 ml) natural soy yogurt or coconut yogurt
4 tablespoons grated celeriac
3 tablespoons sultanas and/or dried physalis
1 tablespoon chia seeds (optional)
1 tablespoon smooth or whole-grain mustard
$^1/_2$ tablespoon probiotic powder, like Udo's (optional)

Serves 2 for lunch or 3 as a side

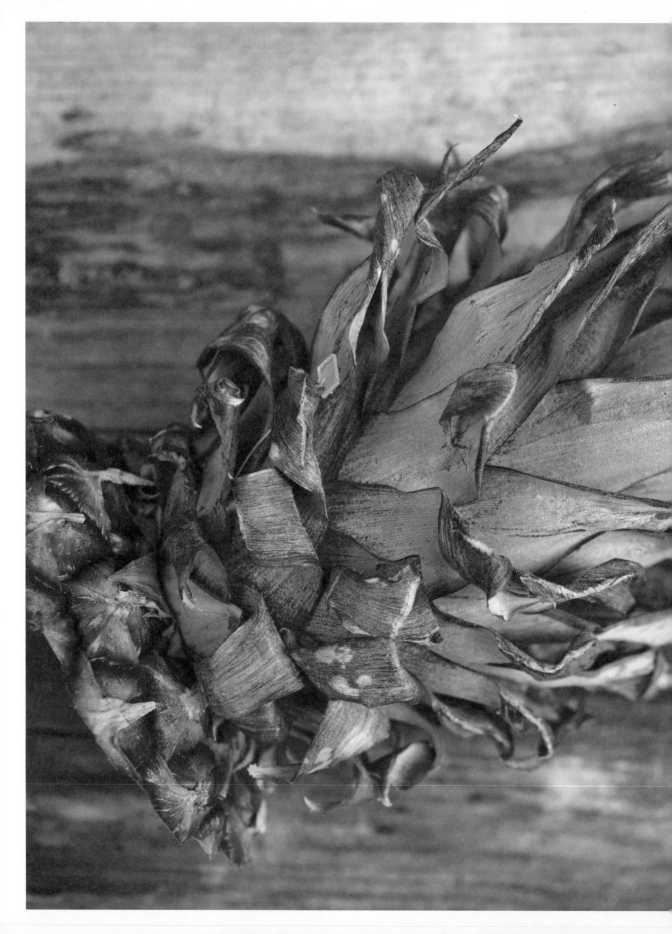

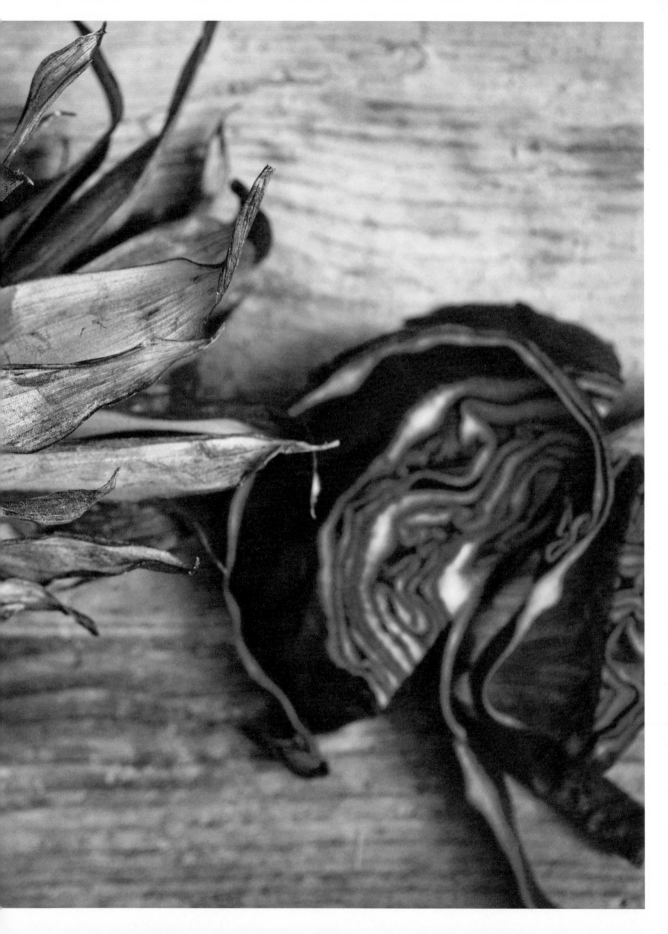

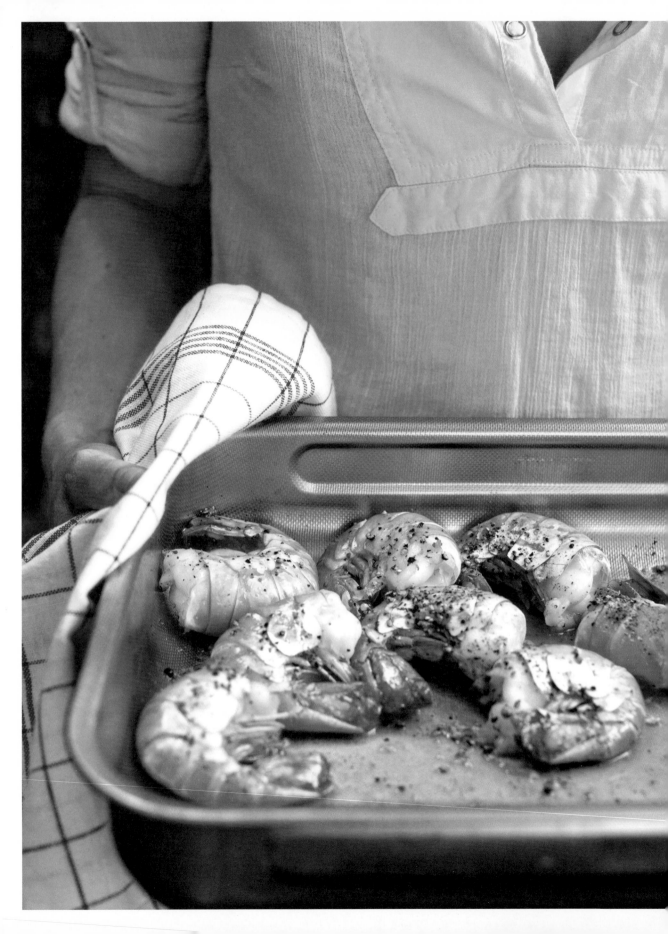

CURRIED CAULI, BANANA, AND SPINACH WITH FLAKED FISH

○○○

Use any fish you like, but I find salmon, mackerel, hake, and cod easiest to flake. Prawns work deliciously well and can be thrown in a hot oven on a separate roasting tray from the cauli. Pan-fried squid is quickest-only ninety seconds to flash-fry in a little extra virgin coconut oil. Ask the fishmonger to prep your squid into rings for you.

Jack up the oven to 410°F (210°C).

Find your biggest roasting tray and briefly melt the oil in it in the oven for a few moments.

Meanwhile, split your cauliflower in half and break into clumsy chunks. Peel and chop the blackened bananas. Remove your roasting tray from the oven, tumble in the cauli, banana, curry powder, and turmeric, and coat everything really well. Roast for 20-25 minutes, shaking from time to time if you remember to. When the cauliflower starts to char, she's done. Remove the tray and mix through the baby spinach.

Meanwhile, to cook the fish, dot a large piece of aluminum foil with coconut oil or your favorite oil. Place the hake or cod on top, then fold the edges of the foil toward each other and seal them together, leaving lots of air above the fish. The fish will steam naturally in this "tent" as long as both sides are sealed. Bake in the same oven as the cauliflower for 15 minutes, until the flesh can be pulled away. It's easy to overcook fish-I find the alarm on my phone to be a good ally in the kitchen. Once you reckon the fish is cooked, remove from its foil tent, season well, and sprinkle with extra spices if you fancy. Set aside until the cauli is ready.

To serve, flake your hake or cod on top of the tray of cauliflower and add a little squeeze of lemon or lime if you have it.

3 tablespoons extra virgin coconut oil
1/2 large head of cauliflower
2 blackened, overripe bananas
3 tablespoons Indian curry powder
1-2 teaspoons ground turmeric (optional for color and nutrition)
Handful of baby spinach leaves
1 large fillet of hake or cod, bones removed
Salt and pepper
Squeeze of lemon or lime juice (optional)

Serves 3

BEGINNER'S BUCKWHEAT WITH GRATED APPLE, CHILI, AND PUMPKIN SEEDS

Instead of boring pasta, which often tastes more like soggy Kleenex than good-quality wheat, give buckwheat a shot. It's a teeny triangular grain, confused by shades of red, brown, and green. The all-familiar Japanese soba noodles and Russian blini are made from buckwheat. Chances are you already like its nutty flavor.

Despite its name, buckwheat is not wheat. Hollywood's glitterati love its slow-release carbs and avalanche of beautifying bioflavonoids. Buckwheat even has lysine, that elusive amino acid responsible for preventing outbreaks of cold sores.

More good news? Once you have the ingredients sourced, this dish takes a mere twelve minutes to rustle up from package to plate.

A handy habit is to store fresh ginger, skin peeled, in your freezer so you never run out of it. Then, with the part of the grater that you normally use for zesting lemons, grate the ginger straight from frozen. Fresh ginger can be a little fibrous, overpowering, and stringy. Frozen ginger is not.

$^1/_4$ cup (35 g) pumpkin seeds

$^1/_2$ teaspoon chili flakes

1 cup (100 g) whole buckwheat grain, rinsed

2 red apples, grated

Up to 1 cup (135 g) gooey, dark, dried apricots, chopped

Splash of extra virgin sesame oil

Good lump of fresh ginger, peeled and frozen (see note above)

Lime juice, to serve

Tamari, to serve

Dried nori flakes, to serve

Serves 4 as a side

Toast the pumpkin seeds with the chili flakes by heating a dry frying pan or wok over a flame and listening for the pumpkin seeds to start popping. Stir briskly and remove when they look pregnant and crispy. Try not to let the pan smoke on high heat.

Bring 1$^1/_2$ cups seasoned water to a boil. Reduce the heat to a rolling simmer, add the freshly rinsed buckwheat, and cook with a lid on for 8-10 minutes, until all the water has been absorbed. Turn off the heat and let the grain steam with the lid on for another few minutes. It should have a bite to it but not a crunch. Drain any excess liquid and rinse with cold water.

Toss the buckwheat with the toasted pumpkin seeds, grated apple, chopped apricots, a splash of sesame oil, and plenty of grated ginger. Serve with a squeeze of lime if you have one or a trickle of tamari and dried nori flakes.

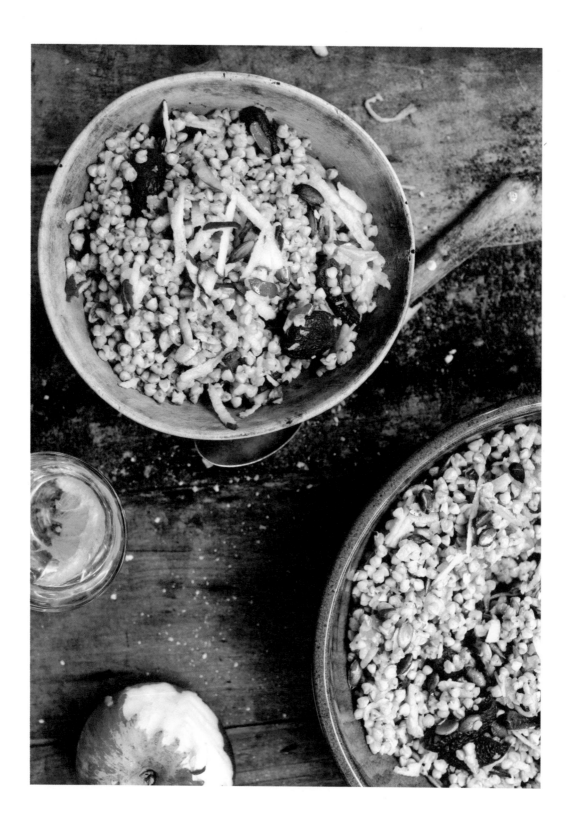

Suppers

One month of eating like this will have you feeling like you're plugged into an electrical socket.

Cooking has never been just about the recipes. It's about navigating
your creativity and flirting with flavors. It's about sensuality
as much as science. To me, it's the ultimate form of self-expression,
where you set out to nourish your body and those you love.

Self-love is distilled in healthy eating. Feeding your body
with nutrient-rich food is like plugging into an electrical socket.
It has the ability to transform energy levels and resurrect brain
cells. Athletes see food as their body's artillery.
It's probably about time we did too. Processed food has little
nutritional purchase, leaving the body bereft of the vital nutrients
necessary for us to function well. Think three-toed sloth or puma:
which would you prefer?

So how can you clean up your diet without losing your personality or
taste buds? It's easier than you think. Here are a couple of tips.

Get your hands on a copy of Wham!'s greatest hits.
I'm not sure if their groove transfers to my fingers,
but something cosmic happens to my serotonin and my pies.
Turn up the volume and get jiggy with it.

Next step is to share the results of your kitchen adventures with
friends. Everyone loves to be fed. There's no easier way of getting
hooked on a new habit than receiving rampant adulation.

The more you surround yourself with healthy people, the more you
start to think like them. I subscribe to great blogs to
get ideas for healthy eating in my inbox every week.
Think of it as a form of helpful "advertising." Cleaning up your diet
may seem slow in the beginning, but persistence will make way for
a new and better you. Just think: if you make one of my recipes every
week, you'll have mastered 52 seriously healthy dishes
by this time next year. Your body is sure to levitate. Ready?

BROWN RICE AND HIS COUSINS

xxxxxxxxxxxxxxxxxxxxxxxxxxxxxxxxxxxxxxxxxxxx

At one stage, American actress Mariel Hemingway made brown rice
so fashionable that Californian grocers struggled to keep it in stock.
Mariel is a bit of a beaut, so it's hardly surprising to find
brown rice, lentils, and chickpeas at the heart of her diet.

You see, whole grains like brown rice contain those mighty B vitamins
responsible for fueling our batteries and busy bods. Vitamin B3
in particular can help lift your mood, like daydreaming about Bradley
Cooper or making small changes to politicians' Wikipedia pages.
There's far less B3, fiber, and manganese in the white starchy stuff.
We need fiber to service our pipes and regulate our poops. Nothing sexy
about constipation. Manganese seems crucial to an antioxidant enzyme
called SOD, the maestro of all antioxidants. One cup of brown rice
delivers almost 100 percent of our daily manga-needs!
Manganese comes from the Greek word for magic. Nuff said.

There are legions of whole-grain rice to choose from; here are
the best ones. Soaking rice apparently improves digestibility and
shortens cooking time. There's no downside to soaking rice,
so it's probably a sensible thing to do.

I use my rice cooker all the time. Exact cooking times and
instructions are on my blog: www.susanjanewhite.com.

Wild rice

Very expensive, so
it's advisable to add
1 tablespoon into other
varieties of rice instead
of serving it straight.
Cooks in 45 minutes.

Brown jasmine rice

Rinse. Simmer 2 parts
water to just over 1
part rice and a pinch of
salt. Follow the direc-
tions on the packet, but
30-40 minutes should be
just about right. Brown
jasmine rice usually takes
less time to cook than
long-grain rice. During
the final few minutes of
cooking, remove the lid
and boil off any remaining
water.

Brown basmati rice

This is the fastest brown
rice to cook. Rinse and
simmer 1 cup brown basmati
with $1^3/_4$ cups seasoned
water. Ready in 22 minutes
(check the cooking time
suggested by the
manufacturer on the
packet). Add 1 teaspoon
of caraway seeds for a
smack of Bombay.

Brown long-grain rice

Most popular but least
impressive. Simmer 2 parts
water to 1 part rice.
You can add 1 tablespoon
of millet, quinoa, wild
rice, or amaranth to 1 cup
of brown long-grain rice
and cook for 45 minutes.
It will be stickier
than regular long-grain
rice but very nourishing
alongside a curry or stew.

Short-grain rice

Rinse. Simmer 2 parts
seasoned water to 1 part
rice. Ready in 45 minutes.
Soaking rice apparently
improves digestibility
and shortens cooking
time. I often do $1^1/_2$ cups
short-grain rice with $^1/_2$
cup whole barley in the
rice cooker. Works beautifully.

Sticky brown sushi rice

Wash sushi rice very well
in cold water. Transfer to
a saucepan with $1^3/_4$ cups
cold water to 1 cup sushi
rice. Soak for 30 minutes,
then boil for 35 minutes.
Remove from the heat and
leave to dry-steam until
all the water is absorbed.
It's best to use a plastic
spatula to avoid splitting
the grain and mushing it.

Red (camargue) rice

Good for beginners. Rinse
and simmer in 2 parts
seasoned water to just
under 1 part rice for
40-50 minutes. Be watchful
of the final few minutes to
avoid burning.

Sweet brown rice

My absolute favorite. It's
a cross between sticky
white rice and short-grain
brown rice. Rinse. Simmer
1 part rice to 2 parts
water. Cook for 35 minutes
or until all the water is
absorbed. Remove from the
heat and allow to dry-steam
with the lid on for a
further 10 minutes.

EGGY FRIED RICE

xxxxxxxxxxxxxxxxxxxxxxx

Every time you make rice, try to remember to make enough for this meal the following day. Then you can high-five your genius when you come home from work and spend 90 seconds whizzing up your supper.

Black garlic keeps for a year in the fridge and is useful for days when you can't dart to the grocer's for fresh stuff. In fact, most of these ingredients will already be lurking in your kitchen. And therein lies its USP.

There's a knack to good fried rice. The first is to cook the eggs completely before adding the rice. The second is never to add soy sauce-it should be served alongside the dish instead. Ready? Let's see if we can get this from fridge to plate in 90 seconds.

1 tablespoon extra virgin coconut oil
$^1/_2$ cup (70 g) frozen peas
2 cups leftover rice
3 black or fresh garlic cloves, chopped
Pinch of arame (optional)
Tamari, to serve

Serves 2

Melt the coconut oil on medium heat in your best frying pan. Make sure the heat isn't too high. While the oil is melting, place the peas in a separate bowl and pour boiling water over them.

Crack the eggs into the pan and poke the yolks so they break. Coat the pan with the eggs. Don't scramble or mix them, but allow them to slowly cook through (around 20 seconds). Now add the rice and stir to coat. Drain the peas and pop them in with the garlic. The arame is optional if you have it in your cupboard (this is an ocean veggie that lasts for up to 3 years in the packet, so it's very handy for suppers like this). Arame demands 10 minutes of soaking too, which would hamper our 90-second challenge right now. But it's something to consider for next time.

Plate up once hot and serve with a bottle of tamari.

BUCKWHEAT CRÊPES WITH PINE NUT RICOTTA AND SPINACH

xxxxxxxxxxxxxxxxxxxxxxxxxxxxxxxxxxxxxxxxxxxxxxxxxxxxxxxxxxxxxxxxxxxxxxxxxxx

I never get my fill on Pancake Tuesday, partly because I always forget it's coming— bit like Mother's Day and Visa deadlines. Pancakes are so darn delicious, it's rather puzzling why we don't tuck into them every Tuesday. Why reserve them for one special day a year?

To make the pine nut ricotta, drain the soaked cashews. Whiz everything together in a mini blender or food processor. A hand-held immersion blender won't work— something more powerful is needed. Scoop into a glass jar and top with crushed black peppercorns.

Boil the frozen spinach in ³/₄ inches of water for 5 minutes. Drain thoroughly. Salt and pepper it up. Keep warm in the oven or on top of the stove until the pancakes are ready to rock.

As you cook each crêpe, keep them warm on a wire rack and cover with a tea towel. Aluminum foil will make the crêpes sweat and turn them soggy. At home, I just serve as I go. There's usually a queue of children at my ankles.

When everyone is seated, dish up the pancakes and dot with pine nut ricotta and a generous dollop of spinach.

1 crêpe recipe (page 78)
Two 10 oz (600 g) packages
  frozen spinach

For the pine nut ricotta:
1 cup (150 g) raw cashews,
  soaked overnight
¹/₂ cup (140 g) pine nuts
1-2 garlic cloves
3 tablespoons water
2 tablespoons extra virgin
  olive oil
2 tablespoons lemon juice
³/₄ teaspoon good-quality sea
  salt
A few turns of the black
  pepper mill
1 tablespoon nutritional
  yeast flakes

Makes 8 crêpes

CHILDREN'S STICKY RICE WITH CAULIFLOWER CONFETTI

xxxxxxxxxxxxxxxxxxxxxxxxxxxxxxxxxxxxxxxxxxxxxxxxxxxxxxxxxxxxxxxxxxxx

1 cup cooked short-grain,
  sweet, or brown sushi rice
3 tablespoons cultured
  coconut yogurt
Floret of purple cauliflower

Serves 2

Rice and quinoa can be tricky for children to master. You can make a "glue" by using mashed sweet potato or coconut yogurt to bind it all together. Using a zester or Microplane, grate the purple cauliflower over each bowl of sticky rice to make purple confetti. Cauliflower has never been so cool!

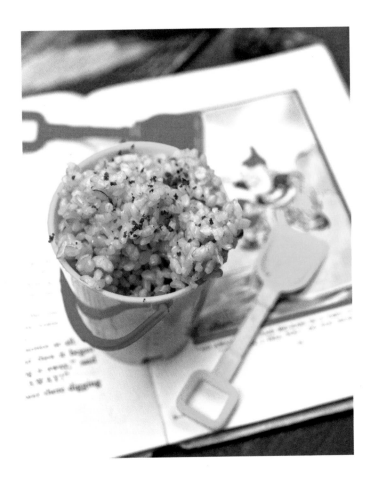

SNAZZY BROCCOLI AND SOBA NOODLES

xxxxxxxxxxxxxxxxxxxxxxxxxxxxxxxxxxxxxxxxxxxxxxxxxxxx

Broccoli is a crusader, backing up your frontline defenses with vitamin C, chloro-phyll, antioxidants, and other handsome phytonutrients. I tell my boys broccoli are edible Lego trees and then they plunder the entire plate.

Famed for its cancer-fighting properties, broccoli is an affordable superfood. When choosing a head, just make sure the florets have not turned yellowish or look limp and tired. With age, broccoli loses those supersonic nutrients.

Cook the soba noodles according to the instructions on the packet. They usually take 8 minutes.

Meanwhile, break the broccoli into bite-size pieces. Steam for 3-4 minutes.

Whisk the garlic with the sesame oil, tamari, Brazil nuts, miso, and cayenne. Reverently drizzle over the warm broccoli, toss with the cooked noodles, and watch your friends and family go bonkers.

1 portion 100% buckwheat soba
 noodles
$1/2$ head of broccoli
2 garlic cloves, crushed
1 tablespoon sesame oil
1 tablespoon tamari
1 tablespoon roughly chopped
 Brazil nuts (optional)
1 teaspoon miso paste
Pinch of cayenne pepper

Serves 2-3

BEGINNER'S QUINOA

*The rapid increase in wheat and gluten sensitivities is good news for quinoa.
This grain practically swaggers with its impressive stash of B vitamins (energy),
protein (repair), iron (strength), magnesium (circulation), and zinc (sexy skin).
Quinoa is really quite the starlet and should be given center stage on your shopping
list. The United Nations' Food and Agriculture Organization considers it to be as
nutritionally complete as whole milk.*

*Quinoa is ideal for picnics and packed lunches, alongside curries, tossed in
salads, scattered into soups, or to accompany a tray of roasted veggies on indolent
evenings.*

1 cup (200 g) quinoa
1¹/₂ cups (375 ml) stock or
  seasoned water
8-12 juicy baby tomatoes,
  halved
Flesh of 1 avocado,
  roughly chopped
1 mild chili, deseeded and
  sliced (optional)
Handful of arugula, chives,
  cress, or cilantro, roughly
  torn
3 tablespoons extra virgin
  olive oil
1 tablespoon finely
  chopped red onion
Sea salt flakes and a few
  twists of the black
  pepper mill

Serves 2

Wash the quinoa very well in a sieve under running water.
Transfer to a heavy-based saucepan. Bring to a boil with
the stock or seasoned water and cook for 12-15 minutes
with a lid on. The longer you cook it, the softer and
stickier it becomes. Take the pan off the heat as soon as
the quinoa has drunk up all the water. Let it sit on the
countertop and fluff up in the residual heat of the lidded
saucepan. Some rice cookers have a special "grain"
setting that works perfectly for quinoa.

Leave the quinoa to cool a little before stirring
through the remaining ingredients. Give the black pepper
mill a few twists and add a smattering of sea salt flakes.
You could pack the quinoa into an empty container for
lunch at the office. I use the cardboard ones from my
local deli's salad counter. They seem far snazzier than
my manky old Tupperware.

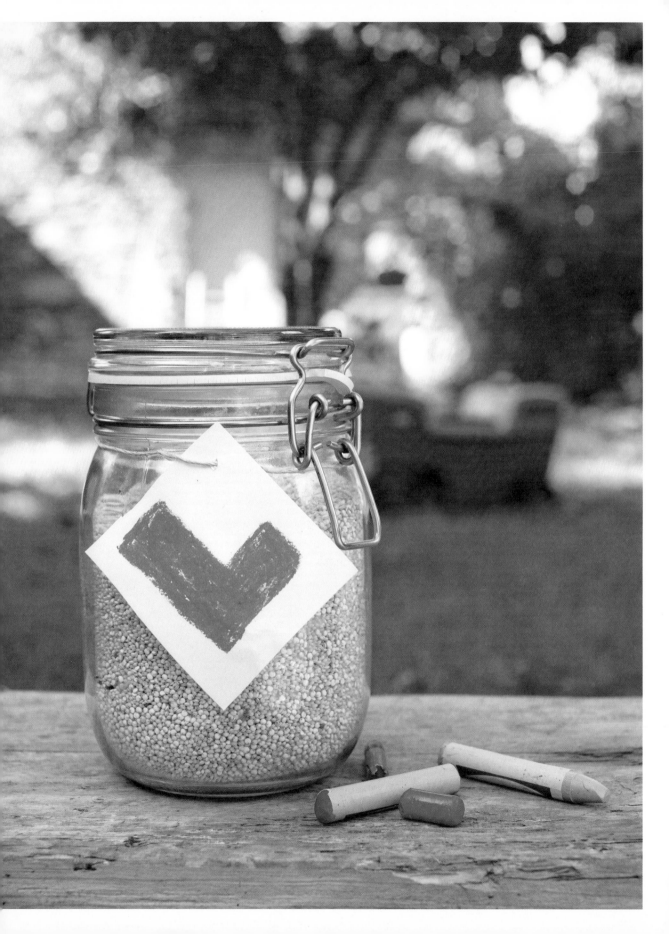

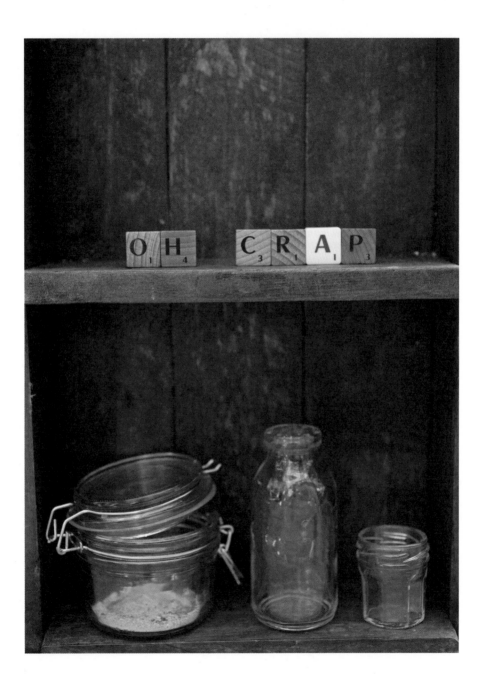

NOTHING-IN-MY-CUPBOARD QUINOA

xxxxxxxxxxxxxxxxxxxxxxxxxxxxxxxxxxxxxxxxxxxxxxx

When the fridge looks bare and you can't find the energy to resuscitate your sleepy brain cells, reach for a packet of quinoa. Uncooked, quinoa will store for ages in your cupboard, making it a very attractive last-minute meal. Here's one to get you started. Cooked quinoa will happily samba in the fridge for a few days.

Soak the arame in water for 10 minutes if using. Drain, and set aside for the quinoa collection. The arame is optional if you have it in your cupboard. Arame is an ocean veggie and lasts for up to 3 years in the packet, so it's very handy for suppers like this.

Thoroughly rinse the quinoa in a sieve under running water. You'll be tempted to skip this step, but try not to or you'll end up with a bitter residue. Drop the rinsed quinoa into your saucepan of boiling salted water. Add the turmeric if you have it and simmer for 12–15 minutes with a lid on it. Drain any excess water from the pan by maneuvering the lid very slightly so that you can pour off the liquid into the sink without losing the heat from the pan. Let the quinoa dry-steam in the saucepan on your countertop for a few more minutes. This step eliminates the threat of soggy quinoa.

When it's done (taste and see), let the quinoa cool a little and toss through the remaining ingredients. The coconut looks better tickled on top. Add as much curry powder as you fancy and a spot of citrus if you feel like it. Olives, capers, pomegranate seeds, and herbs are cracking additions, should you find any loitering in your pantry.

Pinch of arame (optional)
$1^{1}/_{2}$ cups (300 g) quinoa
2 cups (500 ml) seasoned water
1 teaspoon ground turmeric (optional)
$^{1}/_{2}$ cup (75 g) raisins
$^{1}/_{4}$ cup (20 g) desiccated coconut
2 garlic cloves, crushed or minced
1 tall spring onion, sliced
Zest of $^{1}/_{2}$ orange
1 tablespoon Madras curry powder
Good glug of extra virgin olive oil
Smattering of pistachios or any other nut

Serves 3 as a main or 6 as a side

SMOKED PAPRIKA AND CUMIN QUINOA

xxxxxxxxxxxxxxxxxxxxxxxxxxxxxxxxxxxxxxxxxxxxxxxxxxxx

Cooking quinoa is a lot easier than pronouncing it. Insiders call it keen-wah rather than quin-oh-ah, but nobody seems to care what I call it. This curious carb looks and feels the same as couscous, except that it tastes a whole lot nicer. Once you give quinoa a shot, you'll be outraged that couscous ever seduced you.

With its encyclopedic mineral and vitamin profile, quinoa is by far the healthiest grain in my cupboard. It's real fast food with a nutritional halo. Each seed is host to an army of minerals to help service our adrenal glands. These are the call centers for stress and mood. Athletes love quinoa for its low glycemic value. All this means is that a bowl of quinoa can drip-feed your body, brain, and dimples for longer than white bread or pasta. Apparently, it also has higher levels of calcium and protein than dairy. Hail quinoa!

1 cup (200 g) quinoa
1¹/₂ cup (375 ml) hot chicken
  stock or boiling water
2 teaspoons ground cumin
1 teaspoon smoked paprika
2–3 eggs
Generous splash of extra
  virgin olive oil
A few turns of the black
  pepper mill
Bunch of arugula, dill,
  chives, parsley, or
  cilantro

Serves 2–3

Rinse the quinoa in a sieve under running cold water for a good 30 seconds (some grains have a bitter coating). Knock the wet quinoa into a small saucepan. (Bits will stick to the sieve. No matter.) Add the hot chicken stock or boiling water to the quinoa, sprinkle in the spices, and simmer on medium heat for 15 minutes with a lid on. The kitchen will smell incredible. You can tell quinoa is cooked once the tail of the seed comes away from the grain. A nifty trick is to remove the pot from the heat after 12 minutes, drain all the water, and cover the pot with a tightly sealed lid for another 5 minutes. This way, the quinoa won't stick to the base or burn. Any residual heat left in the pot should fluff the grains up nicely.

To poach eggs, make sure you have the freshest eggs possible, left at room temperature, otherwise the eggs may become very disobedient. Using a small heavy-based saucepan, bring 3 inches of water to a simmer. Swirl the water in a circular motion like a whirlpool and slide the raw egg into the middle. Many chefs swear that adding apple cider vinegar to the water will make the egg white behave. Your call. Watch carefully, and remove with a slotted spoon after 60–90 seconds to drain the water off your plump little treasure. Don't worry if it looks like half the egg white is floating in the saucepan. That always happens to me and yet the eggs turn out beautifully.

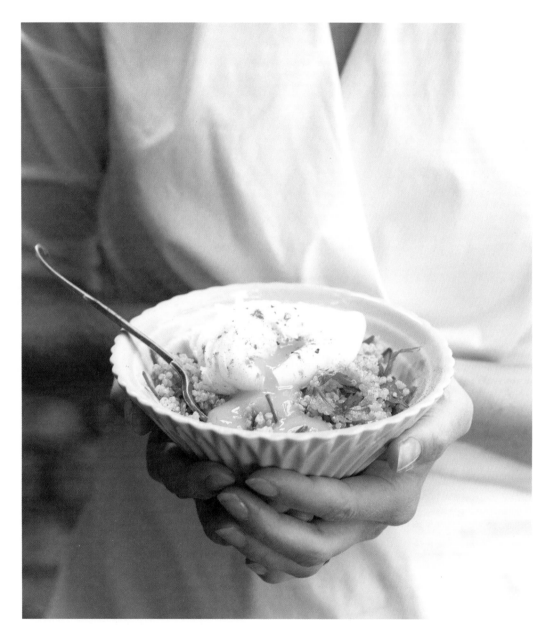

To serve, add a good lick of extra virgin olive oil and a
few turns of the pepper mill to the quinoa. Chop up any
arugula or herbs you can resuscitate from the fridge and
stir them through. Divide between 2 or 3 bowls and crown
with a perfectly poached egg. Poke the egg yolk a little
so its lava oozes out.

HARISSA QUINOA WITH ROASTED LEMON FENNEL

xxxxxxxxxxxxxxxxxxxxxxxxxxxxxxxxxxxxxxxxxxxxxxxxxxxxxxxxxxxx

Harissa is a spicy North African paste guaranteed to send your blood beating like a bodhran. While it looks like a lot of ingredients, you'll find most of them in your cupboard. This should make enough harissa to last 2 weeks in the fridge or 4 months in the freezer.

For the lemon fennel:
4 fennel bulbs
Splash of olive oil
Zest and juice of $1/2$ lemon

For the quinoa:
2 cups (400 g) quinoa, well
    rinsed
3 cups (750 ml) vegetable
    stock or seasoned water

For the harissa:
3-4 red peppers
6 red chilies
4 garlic cloves
1 tablespoon cumin seeds,
    ground
1 tablespoon caraway seeds,
    ground
1 tablespoon smoked paprika
1 tablespoon tomato paste
$1/2$ teaspoon sea salt flakes
1 tablespoon red wine vinegar
3-5 tablespoons extra virgin,
    hemp seed, or olive oil

Serves 4-6

Preheat the oven to 350°F (180°C).

Cut each fennel bulb lengthwise into quarters. Don't be tempted to slice the bum off, as the bulb will fall apart and you will be left with loads of bitty pieces rather than thick wedges. Throw onto a large baking tray.

Now slice the red peppers for the harissa into chunks, discarding the inner white film, stalk, and seeds. Toss on the baking tray with the fennel and a splash of olive oil. Roast for 30 minutes.

While the peppers and fennel cook, bring the quinoa and stock to a rolling boil. Reduce the heat until it's puttering away politely. Put a lid on it and cook for about 12 minutes. Drain (if the stock is not thoroughly absorbed), place the lid back on, and let the grains fluff up from the residual heat of the saucepan for another 5 minutes.

While the quinoa and roasted veggies do their thing, let's get going on the fresh harissa. Wearing disposable gloves, cut the chilies down the side and scoop out the seeds and pith with a teaspoon. Discard. Or rub on husband's toothbrush if he hasn't taken out the trash. Blitz the chilies with the garlic, spices, tomato paste, and salt until it forms a smooth paste. I find a hand-held blender much better than a food processor for this. Now, and no sooner, add the roasted red peppers (pick them out from the tray of roasted fennel) and the vinegar. Pulverize to your satisfaction. Stir through the hemp oil or olive oil and scoop into your serving dish. Avoid adding the oil while pulverizing the rest of the ingredients or the harissa will turn pink and no one will eat it, not even your Barbie-loving toddler.

To serve the whole lot, gloss up the quinoa with a smidge
of olive oil. Divide between 4-6 plates, top with a
couple of fennel wedges, the zest and juice of a little
lemon, and a royal dollop of harissa.

QUINOA WITH STRAWBERRY AND MINT GREMOLATA

xxxxxxxxxxxxxxxxxxxxxxxxxxxxxxxxxxxxxxxxxxxxxxxxxxxxxxxxxxxxx

This is the kind of dish that will make you purer simply by looking at it. If you haven't cooked quinoa before, it's the perfect food for taking into work and dining al desko. Bring an extra fork to ward off envious colleagues forced to queue for manky cafeteria food.

If you're worried about evacuating the office at lunchtime with your honking breath, fear not: parsley can help neutralize garlic breath. Crushed walnuts are another stealthy trick to remember. Failing that, peppermint oil capsules from health food stores are a winner and will make you giggle when you have gloriously refreshing burps.

2 cups (400 g) quinoa
3 cups (750 ml) stock or
  seasoned water
1 teaspoon ground turmeric
  (optional for color and
  nutrition)

For the strawberry mint
  gremolata:
2 garlic cloves
1 lemon
$^1/_2$ cup (125 ml) extra virgin
  olive oil
Generous helping of salt
  flakes and crushed black
  pepper
25 g curly parsley
25 g mint leaves
$^1/_4$ cup (25 g) dried
  strawberries (fresh
  won't work)

Serves 2 as a main or 4 as
  a side

Rinse the quinoa under running water for 30 seconds, rubbing the grains together with your fingers. A sieve is helpful. Knock the rinsed quinoa into a saucepan (don't worry about the bits that stick to the sieve; these are designed to test your patience and are destined for the kitchen sink). Add the stock and turmeric. Bring to a rolling boil, lower the heat, and fit a lid on top. Cook for 10–15 minutes, until all the liquid is absorbed. You'll know it's cooked as soon as you see a little tail on each grain. If you like it soft, keep the lid on and let it dry-steam on the counter for a further 5–10 minutes. This will make the grain nice and fluffy without the risk of burning.

To make the strawberry mint gremolata while the quinoa cooks, finely grate the garlic and lemon rind. Squeeze a tiny bit of juice from the lemon into a jam jar and add the olive oil, salt, and pepper. Chop the parsley and mint into it. Give everything a jolly good mix in the jar by shaking it all wildly.

Let the quinoa cool a little before dressing it up. I find hot quinoa always absorbs more than I'd like it to, resulting in disappointing, squidgy quinoa. When it feels cooler, tumble in the dressing and dried strawberries.

KATE MOSS QUINOA

xxxxxxxxxxxxxxxxxxxxxxxxx

Every time I eat quinoa, I feel like a supermodel. This elegant grain contains around 17 percent complete protein, making it white-hot for vegans, athletes, and professional nuts (nutritionists). Celebs love the stuff. Bloggers are possessed by it. And overpriced restaurants have hijacked its pulling power with an excitement usually reserved for a Disney premiere. This grain is going places.

Quinoa is perfect to bring in for lunch at the office. Black+Blum sell dinky bento boxes and lunch sets online (see page 253).

Rinse the quinoa under cold running water for at least 30 seconds, using your fingers to rub the grains together. Plonk the now-wet grain into a small saucepan and add the stock and turmeric. Bring to boiling point, cover with a lid, turn down the heat slightly, and cook for 12 minutes, until all the liquid has been soaked up. Remove from the heat and allow the saucepan to stand on the kitchen counter for a further 5 minutes with the lid on. This step is important if you like fluffy quinoa. Taste and decide for yourself. As soon as you're happy with it, let the grain cool down (I spread it out on a large flat plate).

While your quinoa is puttering away, prep the remaining ingredients. Slice the red onion in half and thinly shave into semicircles using a sharp knife. Soak in the red wine vinegar for 15 minutes. Cut the pomegranate into quarters and peel back the white pith to reveal lots of ruby-red seeds. You're aiming for about 1/4 cup of pomegranate seeds.

In a large bowl, add the pom seeds, blueberries, dill, garlic, and olive oil. I recommend using 8 cloves of creamy roasted garlic and mashing them into a paste with the oil. Drain the red onion before adding it to the remaining ingredients (you'll need to discard the vinegar).

Once you're satisfied with the texture of your quinoa, add to your prepped ingredients and give it a nice tumble and tickle. Crown with extra blueberries, or lamb cutlets for carnivores.

1 cup (200 g) quinoa
1 1/2 cups (375 ml) vegetable stock or seasoned water
1/4 teaspoon ground turmeric
1 small red onion
3 tablespoons red wine vinegar
1 small pomegranate
Handful of blueberries
1 bunch (30 g) of dill, stems removed
1 clove freshly minced garlic or 8 cloves roasted garlic (see page 94)
4 tablespoons extra virgin olive oil

Serves 2 as a main or 5 as a side

CHILDREN'S QUINOA

xxxxxxxxxxxxxxxxxxxxxxxxxxx

Quinoa is a carb indigenous to Peru. As a grain, it's sort of like couscous, only nuttier in taste and significantly healthier. Quinoa provides essential amino acids that the body requires for optimum functioning, making it a first-class plant protein. No wonder those wily Peruvians can skip up the Incan altitudes with the ease of greyhounds at a marathon. My children love the stuff.

Quinoa is even powdered down and sold in capsule form, such is its nutritional bounty. This children's recipe has a stash of other immune-enhancing superfoods, such as sweet potato, mango, goji berries, virgin coconut oil, and turmeric. No nursery bug will stand a chance!

1 cup (200 g) quinoa
1¹/₂ cups (375 ml) filtered
  water or chicken stock
2 tablespoons goji berries
  (optional nutrition)
1 teaspoon ground turmeric
2 tablespoons extra virgin
  coconut oil
1 sweet potato, baked.whole
¹/₂ mango (optional nutrition)

Serves 2-4

Rinse the quinoa very well under running water. A sieve is useful. Knock the wet quinoa grains into a saucepan (don't worry about the bits that stick to the sieve; these are designed to test your patience and are destined for the kitchen sink). Add the water, goji berries (if using), and turmeric. Bring to a rolling boil, lower the heat, and fit a lid on top. Cook for 12-15 minutes, until all the liquid is absorbed. You'll know it's cooked as soon as you see a little tail on each grain. Children like it soft, so keep the lid on and let it dry-steam on the counter for a further 10 minutes. This will make the grain nice and fluffy without the risk of burning. Add the coconut oil and replace the lid.

Peel and roughly mash the baked sweet potato (it won't matter what size it is). Finely chop the mango. Mix into the fluffy quinoa. The mash acts like a glue to bind the quinoa together, making it easier for children to eat.

BASIC LENTILS

Heart disease is the world's biggest killer, chased closely by bowel cancer.
If you're worried about either condition, make friends with your health insurer.
Or lentils. You don't have to be a member of the Green Party to enjoy them or start
campaigning against animal cruelty. Just a little mustard and garlic, and in no time
you'll be the best of friends.

Lentils are the heavyweight champion of fiber. Why is this important to you? Fiber
helps maintain a healthy cholesterol range by deporting excess bile from the body.
The lower your cholesterol range, the lower your risk of heart disease (CVD, in
doctor speak). At the same time, fiber gives your pipes a first-rate servicing. A cup
of lentils holds a stonking 17 grams of fiber. That's more than half our recommended
daily intake. These tiny legumes have other salubrious gifts for your ticker, such
as potassium and magnesium. See ya later, paltry pasta!

The Blue Zones Diet, also dubbed the Centenarian's Diet, is a compilation of foods
we should be paying close attention to if we are planning to cavort well into our
nineties. The diet reveals how centenarians across the world manage to live longer
and better and still look buff at ninety-nine without pills or Crème de la Mer.
And you know what? Beans and lentils are among their top foods. Here are a few good
recipes to bring into the office with you. Lentils love dining al desko.

Simmer the lentils gently with a lid on for 15-20 minutes (if you're using Canadian or brown lentils, they'll need more water and an extra 10-15 minutes). Lentils are cooked when they look like they're yawning. A bit like mussels, only 20 times smaller. Puy lentils cook rapidly and hold their shape very well compared to other varieties.

Try not to add salt until afterward, or the lentils' skin can toughen. Once cooked, or when the cooking liquid has evaporated, lick with extra virgin olive oil, raw apple cider vinegar, and a smattering of celery salt. They're not very demanding.

1 cup (210 g) Puy lentils
1¹/₂ cups (375 ml) stock or water
Extra virgin olive oil
Raw apple cider vinegar
Celery salt

Serves 2

MAPLE MUSTARD LENTILS

xxxxxxxxxxxxxxxxxxxxxxxxxxxxxxx

1 Basic Lentils recipe (page
157)

For the dressing:
1 small garlic clove, crushed
3 tablespoons extra virgin
olive oil
2 tablespoons balsamic or
raw apple cider vinegar
1-2 teaspoons maple syrup
1 tablespoon smooth Dijon
mustard
1 teaspoon black or mixed
peppercorns, crushed
Handful of salad leaves or
fresh herbs

Serves 2 as a side

Cook the lentils as outlined on page 157. Combine all
the dressing ingredients (except the herbs) before
pouring over the warm lentils and then stirring
through some herbs. A great side plate to fish and
meat. My husband and I tend to add finely chopped
anchovies to ours, but I realize not everyone shares
our anchovy fetish.

Leftover dressing can be refrigerated in a clean jam
jar for 2 weeks.

PUMPKIN AND BLACK GARLIC LENTILS

xxxxxxxxxxxxxxxxxxxxxxxxxxxxxxxxxxxxxxxxxxxxxxxx

1 small organic pumpkin
Extra virgin coconut or olive
oil
1 Basic Lentils recipe
(page 157)
6 cloves of black aged garlic,
finely sliced
A couple of anchovies,
finely sliced (optional)
Coconut yogurt, to serve

Serves 6 as a side

Preheat the oven to 425°F (220°C).

Quarter the pumpkin using a sharp knife (and even
sharper concentration-no one wants roasted fingers).
Deseed the flesh and roughly chop into 2-inch pieces-
no need to peel the skin. Splash with coconut or olive
oil and make sure everything is well coated. Roast
on a baking tray for 45 minutes, shaking the tray
halfway through the cooking time. Remove the pumpkin
once the sides start to caramelize. Tumble into the
cooked lentils and sprinkle with the black garlic
and anchovies (if using). Tuck your creation into a
lunch carton, ready to pack into your briefcase the
next day. Try not to scoff it all at the bus stop in the
morning or you'll weep at lunchtime.

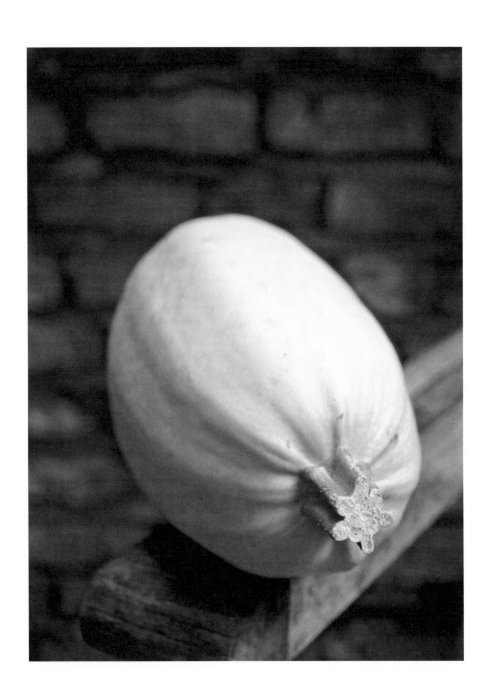

CANNED SARDINES FIVE WAYS

XXXXXXXXXXXXXXXXXXXXXXXXXXXXXXXXXXXXXXXXX

Canned sardines are an excellent source of omega-3, calcium, protein, and vitamin D. Let's not go into bone density here, but suffice it to say that if you want to groove on the dance floor well into your sixties, get 'em in ya! There ain't nothing sexy about brittle bones. Here are a couple of ideas to get you foxtrotting with sardines again.

Chermoula-Kissed Sardines

This North African chermoula has been Irishified with a touch of seaweed. Arame requires only a little soaking before it's ready to dance. Don't be afraid of using seaweed in your cuisine-it's easier than opening a can of beans!

Good pinch of arame
4 garlic cloves
1 teaspoon whole black peppercorns
1 cup flat-leaf parsley, chopped
1 cup cilantro, chopped
$^1/_2$ cup (125 ml) extra virgin olive oil
2 tablespoons ground cumin
2 tablespoons lemon juice
$^1/_2$ teaspoon cayenne pepper

Soak the arame in water for 10 minutes while you prep the other ingredients.

Crush the garlic and peppercorns in a mortar. Briskly stir in the remaining ingredients with a fork. This is tradi-tional chermoula.

Drain the arame and discard the soaking liquid. Finely chop and stir through the chermoula. Moroccans love it on hardboiled eggs or white fish, or tumbled into chickpeas. I think it's cosmic with sardines.

Smoky Sardines

Drain the canned sardines. Mash with crushed garlic and a good pinch of smoked paprika. Serve on top of half an avocado.

Mediterranean Sardines

Drain the canned sardines and mash with chopped sun-dried tomatoes, olives, parsley, and lemon zest. Tastes great on dehydrated flaxseed crackers if you can find them. My boys eat these every week.

Balsamic Sardines

Drain the sardines of their oil or brine and combine with a splash of balsamic vinegar and chopped chives (or any herb from your window farm). Use celery stalks and red pepper strips as edible spoons.

Curried Mayo and Sardines

You can make your own curried mayo using health-enhancing oils (see page 48 and add 3 tablespoons of curry powder at the beginning). The mayo will last for 3 weeks in the fridge. Just reach for a can of sardines and crown on top of a simple salad of romaine lettuce leaves and chopped apple. Go for papaya or mango if you're dead fancy.

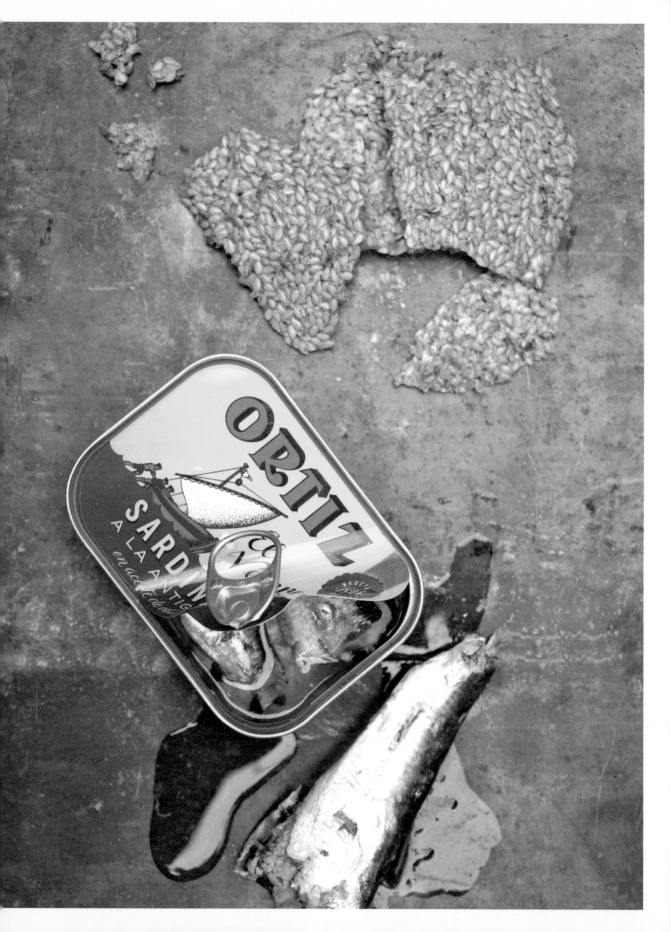

MACKEREL PÂTÉ WITH ANCHOVY AIOLI

xxxxxxxxxxxxxxxxxxxxxxxxxxxxxxxxxxxxxxxxxxxxxx

This is the short-top-and-sides of evening meals.

It's clear we need to look for sustainable fish if we want our grandchildren's kids to know what tuna and salmon taste like. Overfishing is leading to extinction. Our choices affect real-time demand in the marketplace, and fishing is a demand-driven industry. If you're unsure, look for the Marine Stewardship Council (MSC) label of approval.

Mackerel is on tap in Ireland. It has to be the tastiest, cheapest, and most plentiful fish I can get my greedy mitts on. If gutting or filleting fresh fish is too much for your blood pressure, ask Mr. Terribly Kind Fishmonger to do it for you.

2 hardboiled eggs
1 large fillet cooked/smoked
  mackerel or one 4.41 oz
  (125 g) can of mackerel
3 tablespoons anchovy aioli
  (page 48) or coconut yogurt
1-2 tablespoons chopped
  spring onion or fresh dill

Serves 2

Pulse the eggs, fish, and aioli or yogurt in a food processor before adding the chopped herbs. Make it as chunky or as smooth as you wish, but don't whiz the herbs or you'll end up with what looks like remnants of Kermit the Frog.

Canned mackerel works best with aioli and smoked mackerel with yogurt. It's great on half an avocado or the Your New Wheat-Free Bread (page 51). Bring leftovers into work the next day in a jar for a sneaky midmorning dining al desko experience. Fishavores might like to alternate mackerel with kippers or canned wild salmon and capers.

BAKED HAKE WITH LEMONGRASS SALSA

xxxxxxxxxxxxxxxxxxxxxxxxxxxxxxxxxxxxxxxxxxxxxxxxxxxx

Farmers know all about the importance of nutrient-rich soil to grow top-quality produce. It's no different for us-nourish your body and your body will nourish you.

With that in mind, get your entire five a day with this mango and lemongrass salsa. It's also ace to bring to a BBQ. Word of caution-this salsa is the prima donna of accompaniments, made to outshine all others. Your host will hate you.

Preheat the oven to 400°F (200°C).

Season the hake with salt and pepper and place on a piece of aluminum foil. Secure into a tent-like parcel, transfer the tent onto a baking tray, and cook for approximately 15 minutes. I always dot the fish with extra virgin coconut oil and a splash of mirin or ume, but you decide. The basic message I want to convey is that cooking fish is easy peasy. The razzmatazz is up to you.

You'll know it's cooked when it falls apart with pressure from your thumb. Raw fish won't. While the hake bakes, get going on your salsa.

There's no need to peel your mango straightaway. Using a sharp knife, slice down either side of its flat, oblong stone. Cut each slice into 5 or 6 strips. Similar to a slice of melon, run your knife along the skin of each strip of mango to free its flesh. Lick your fingers and chop into small chunks. The mango, not your fingers. Peel the ginger, discarding its gnarly skin, and freeze its core for 15 minutes. Freezing fresh ginger makes it easier to grate straight into salads.

Gently toss all the salsa ingredients together. Remove the ginger from the freezer and grate it over the salsa.

When your hake is happy, serve on a big plate with the salsa running over the fish. It will end up like a large cross on the plate-the idea is not to hide the fish under the salsa. If you have any black olives lurking in your cupboards, scatter a couple over the fish for a touch of *Mary Poppins*.

1 large piece of hake
A few turns of the salt and
  peppercorn mill

For the salsa:
1 mango
Thumb-sized piece of fresh
  ginger
1 cup cherry tomatoes,
  quartered
3 spring onions, chopped
1 red chili, deseeded and
  sliced into circles
1 lemongrass stalk, white
  part finely minced
$1/3$ cucumber, cut into small
  chunks
Handful of chopped cilantro
Juice and zest of 1 lime
Decent glug of extra virgin
  olive oil

Serves 2

SIMPLE SALMON WITH ASPARAGUS SOLDIERS AND WHIPPED GREEN TEA

xxxxxxxxxxxxxxxxxxxxxxxxxxxxxxxxxxxxxxxxxxxxxxxxxxxxxxxxxxxxxxxxxxxxxxxxxxxxxxxxxxxxxxxxx

The latest research on folic acid is rather titillating. Sufficient quantities of this B vitamin can help prolong sexual orgasms. I wonder who signed up for those trials. And whether those in the placebo group were just plain boring? Suddenly, folic acid seems as important to my hedonistic rights as my favorite chocolate pie.

Where can we stock up on this much-coveted substance? Your local grocery store. Asparagus is full of folate (folic acid). That's why they call it vegans' Viagra.

2 salmon or trout fillets
  (certifiably sustainable
  if possible)
Dot of extra virgin coconut
  or sesame oil
Large bunch of asparagus
2 tablespoons toasted
  sesame oil

For the whipped green tea:
Flesh of 1 large, ripe avocado
Juice of 1 orange
1 teaspoon wasabi powder
  or paste (Dijon mustard
  will do)
1 teaspoon matcha green tea
Salt and pepper

Serves 2

Preheat the oven to 400°F (200°C).

Prepare the salmon by wrapping the fillets in a parcel of aluminum foil and dotting with the oil. I use extra virgin raw coconut oil, but use whatever you're happiest with. Make sure there's lots of space above the fillets—it's more like a tent than a parcel. This way the fish steams in its own juices.

Transfer the tent of salmon onto a baking tray and roast for 10-15 minutes, depending on how big the fillets are. Check by pulling the flesh apart. If they're not done, just reseal your tent and pop them in the oven again. When you've become familiar with this method of cooking, crank it up another level by adding smashed lemon-grass, maple syrup, chili, cumin, kaffir lime leaves, or whatever tickles your appetite on any given evening.

To roast the asparagus, start by removing the tougher ends of each asparagus spear. Gently bend each spear until it snaps. Trust the vegetable—it's sort of like natural selection. Discard the stalky parts and tumble the tender heads in a baking tray with the sesame oil. Roast for 10-15 minutes (same as the salmon tents), which should make them tender but not squishy.

To make the whipped green tea, give the avocado, orange juice, wasabi, matcha, and a touch of seasoning a jolly fine whiz with a hand-held blender. That's all there is to it. Taste, and add more wasabi if you need to ignite a dull evening or a vexatious guest.

Smear your dinner plates with a generous serving of
the whip and place a fillet on top. You can arrange the
asparagus on top of the salmon Jenga-style if you're
brave enough.

SALMON FISH CAKES WITH CURRIED COCONUT YOGURT

xxxxxxxxxxxxxxxxxxxxxxxxxxxxxxxxxxxxxxxxxxxxxxxxxxxxxxxxxxxxxxxxxxxx

Wild salmon is the Tom Brady of the ocean: indecently tasty and hard to catch. Not bad for the heart and circulation either.

This supersonic fish is hailed for its cargo of omega-3, vitamin D, and niacin. But before I get too misty eyed about the benefits of eating salmon, I should stress that not all salmon "products" are created equal. Smoked, canned, farmed, or wild—each has a different nutritional purchase. While smoked might be the tastiest and the most popular, its canned counterpart offers a lot more calcium without the smoky nitrates. Nitrates are under the watchful eye of food scientists, given their possible correlation to an increased risk of certain cancers. But then, we also have to temper our love of canned food with questions hanging over the chemicals used in the cans. Put down the iPhone. Nothing to tweet about. Just something to be aware of should you be gobbling industrial quantities of the stuff.

Then there's the ubiquitous farmed or caged salmon, most of which are fed with dodgy colorings and antibiotics. Some farmers in the United States choose how pink or red they want their salmon from a color wheel called the Salmofan. Nostril-flaring stuff. However, unlike its wilder cousin, farmed salmon is a fraction of the price and available fresh all year round. Two important factors for prudent parents.

So what does the savvy shopper do? Look for organically farmed salmon or Marine Stewardship Council endorsements, eat moderate amounts of the smoked stuff, and flirt with the canned variety from time to time.

These are definitely better and cheaper than any fancy fish cake we've sunk our teeth into at restaurants. You can easily personalize this basic recipe by introducing your favorite spice: try some crushed cumin seeds, nutritional yeast flakes, caraway and fenugreek, cilantro, or pummelled black onion seed.

$1^1/_2$ cups (300 g) lightly
  mashed potatoes
2 spring onions, chopped
1 fillet cooked salmon, flaked
  (see page 164)
1 chili, sliced (not chili
  powder)
1 fat garlic clove, minced
1 small egg, beaten
Zest of $1/_2$ unwaxed lemon
Good hunk of fresh ginger,
  peeled and minced
Generous seasoning
Extra virgin coconut oil,
  for frying

With a fork, stir together the potatoes, spring onions, salmon, chili, garlic, egg, lemon zest, ginger, and salt and pepper.

Heat your frying pan with a blob of extra virgin coconut oil. When your pan is sufficiently hot, drop a heaping spoonful of the fish cake mixture onto the pan, pat with a spatula and turn down the heat a little to prevent it from burning. Cook both sides until lightly colored.

Meanwhile, mix together the yogurt and the curry powder. Serve the fish cakes cold or at room temperature (not

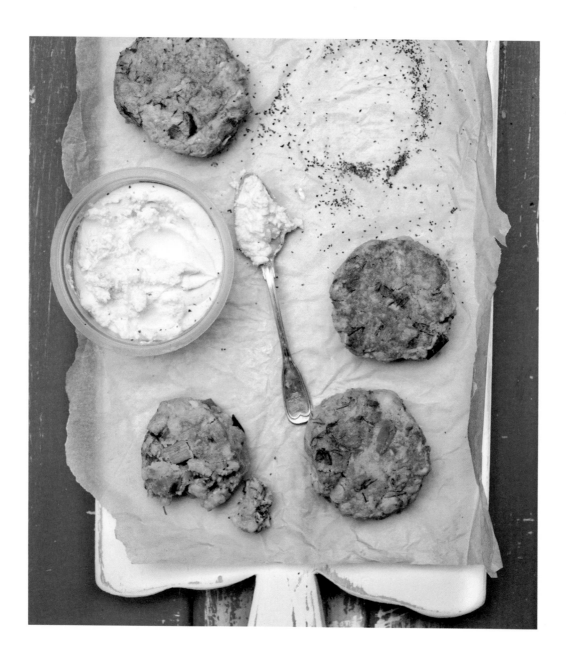

hot) with a dollop of spicy yogurt. The Vietnamese mint dipping sauce on page 170 is pretty special too. Chill them overnight if packing for a sneaky breakfast on the bus to work.

For the curried coconut yogurt:
1 small tub of natural or coconut yogurt
1 tablespoon sweet curry powder

Makes 8 fish cakes

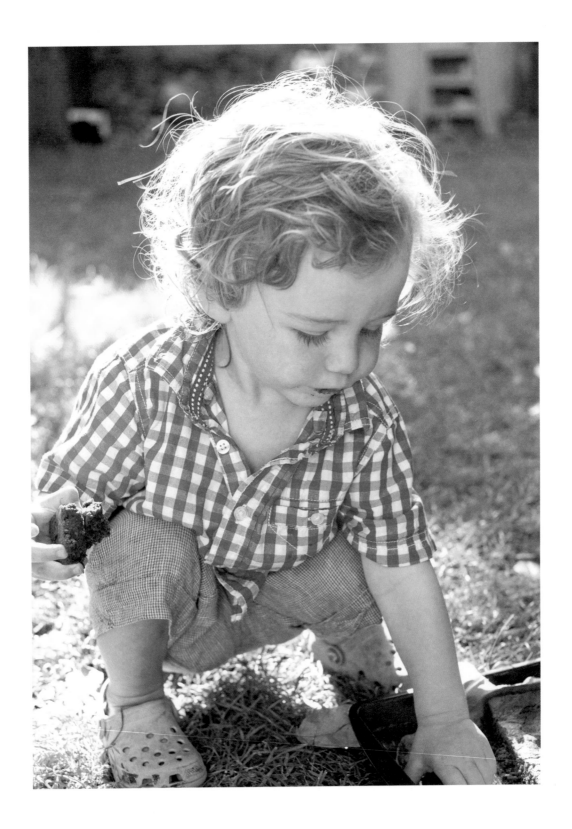

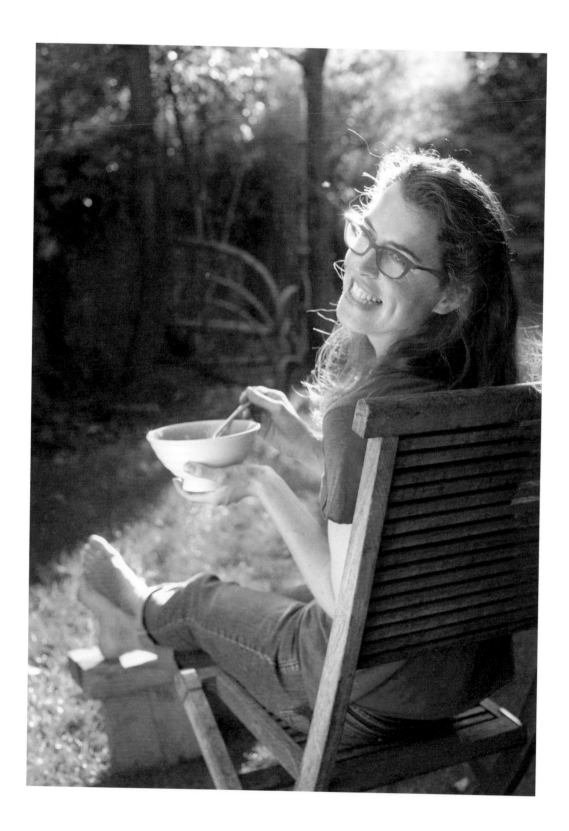

CHIA CRAB CAKES WITH VIETNAMESE MINT DIPPING SAUCE

xxxxxxxxxxxxxxxxxxxxxxxxxxxxxxxxxxxxxxxxxxxxxxxxxxxxxxxxxxxxxxxxxxxxxxx

Chia is an optional lah-di-dah. These teensy seeds deliver a whackload of omega-3 brainpower. But if you can still remember how to solve a polynomial root with the factor theorem, you can probably leave them out.

The Vietnamese dipping sauce will leave a really refreshing taste in your mouth. If you can't be bothered making it, just add some miso paste to the mashed potatoes and wrestle some dill in there too.

For the dipping sauce:
1 red chili, seeds removed
  and finely sliced
Juice of 1 lime
4-6 tablespoons very finely
  chopped mint
1 tablespoon fish sauce
  (nam pla)
1 tablespoon sesame oil
1 tablespoon tamari
1 tablespoon raw honey, agave
  nectar, or yacón syrup

For the crab cakes:
2 tablespoons chopped dried
  mango, soaked overnight
1½ cups (300 g) lightly
  mashed potatoes
½-1 cup (200 g) crabmeat
1 fat garlic clove, crushed
1 tablespoon chia seeds
  soaked in 2 tablespoons
  water
1 teaspoon Szechuan or black
  peppercorns, crushed
Squeeze of lime juice
Generous seasoning
2 tablespoons brown rice
  flour, to dust (optional)
Extra virgin coconut oil,
  for frying
Bean sprouts, to serve
Little Gem lettuces, to serve

Makes 10 small crab cakes

To make the dipping sauce, whisk everything together. Honey can be sticky, but don't worry, it eventually submits.

To make the crab cakes, start by draining the soaked mango pieces. Fresh mango won't work quite as well as its dried equivalent. Using a fork, crush with the remaining crab cake ingredients except the brown rice flour and coconut oil. If you're not making the dipping sauce, be sure to add some miso or nutritional yeast flakes to the mix for oomph. Mold into 10 small crab cakes and dust with brown rice flour (if using).

Heat a large frying pan with a little coconut oil and briefly brown each crab cake. Allow to cool completely before serving, otherwise they'll fall apart in your hands and you'll curse me. Really tasty served alongside bean sprouts and Little Gem lettuce-use the lettuce leaves to scoop up the minty mess.

FISH FINGERS WITH BEETROOT KETCHUP

xxxxxxxxxxxxxxxxxxxxxxxxxxxxxxxxxxxxxxxxxxxxxxxxxxxxxxxxx

Beetroot is still ranked as one of the most underused and misunderstood veggies. It's easy to find in supermarkets, yet it doesn't always mosey its way into our baskets. Dr. Jonny Bowden, nutritional adviser to Hollywood's elite, rates it among his top superfoods. Good news for recessionistas and eco warriors because it's cheap, plentiful, and comes with a low carbon footprint. We make ketchup from it. It goes devastatingly well with a salad of grated carrots, celeriac, pear, and hazelnuts, for example, and keeps very well in the fridge.

You don't have to use nutritional yeast flakes in the crumb coating, but they're seriously handy to have in your cupboard. Dubbed the vegan's Parmesan, yeast flakes give your dish a nutritional upgrade and some real spine. There's also seaweed, which may sound gross but is in fact outrageously healthy. It helps bring the classic fish finger to another cosmos. Without it, they'd only hit the clouds.

These freeze exceptionally well (provided you're not using frozen fillets), so try to double the batch. They're the quickest healthy supper you can have for growing children without breaking into a sweat.

Preheat the oven to 400°F (200°C). Line a baking tray with parchment paper.

To make the beetroot ketchup, dice the beets. If using vacuum-packed beets, ensure there is no vinegar added as a preservative. Purée the ketchup ingredients with a hand-held blender until sumptuously smooth. Adjust the sweetness or sharpness to your preference. The honey or agave will sweeten the ketchup, while apple cider vinegar gives it attitude. A tiny amount of each makes a noticeable difference. Season.

To make the fish fingers, whiz the seaweed, yeast flakes, and lemon zest in a food processor until they are uniform. Now stir through your almonds and transfer the mixture onto a large plate.

On another plate, lay out your chosen flour—rye, quinoa, oat, whatever you have. Pour the beaten egg onto a third plate and put the pieces of fish on a fourth plate. You're ready to rock.

(continued)

For the fish fingers:
$^1/_2$ cup (20 g) mixed dried
  seaweed, finely chopped
$^1/_2$ cup (20 g) nutritional
  yeast flakes (optional)
Zest of 1 lemon (optional)
$2^1/_2$ cups (250 g) ground
  almonds or wheat-free
  breadcrumbs
$^1/_2$ cup (60 g) flour of choice
  (chickpea flour doesn't
  work)
1 large egg, beaten
4 fillets wild salmon,
  pollock, or lemon sole,
  cut into strips

For the beetroot ketchup:
4 medium-size cooked or
  vacuum-packed beets
1 garlic clove, crushed
1 tablespoon apple cider
  vinegar

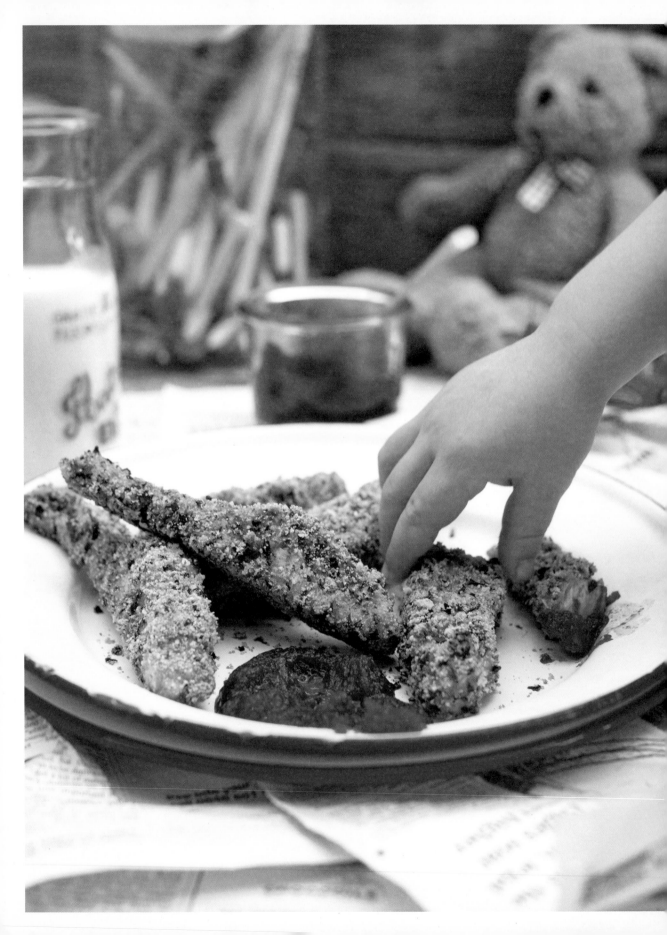

Using a fork-your hands need to be dry-scoop up a piece of fish, dust with flour, dip into the egg and dunk into the crumb coating. That's one fish finger. Settle on the lined baking tray and repeat until all the pieces of fish are coated.

Cook in the oven for 8-16 minutes, depending on the thickness of your fish. Lemon sole will take only 8 minutes, while thicker wedges of fish can take up to 16 minutes. Serve with the beetroot ketchup, a mini bowl of peas, or diced avocado. Seriously snazzy.

1 tablespoon raw honey or
  brown rice syrup
2 teaspoons organic soy or
  coconut yogurt
Salt and pepper

Makes 16-20 fish fingers

CHOPPED HERRING AND THE LAUREATES

xxxxxxxxxxxxxxxxxxxxxxxxxxxxxxxxxxxxxxxxxxxxxxxxxxxxx

This is a classic Jewish recipe. Considering 58 percent of Nobel Prize winners in economics are of Jewish descent, it would be fair to conclude that Jewish mamas know how to nourish their brood.

Mood and activity in the brain are dependent on a series of chemical signals that cross each membrane with the help of neurotransmitters. This intricate process is referred to as transduction-sort of like a messaging service or a call center. Now that we know omega-3 fats are a core component in every cell membrane, they are deemed crucial for signal transduction. In other words, happy call center staff.

If, like me, you'd rather supplement your diet naturally with food and not pharma, then fill your shopping basket with foods rich in omega-3: herring, mackerel, wild salmon, sardines, anchovies, flaxseeds, chia seeds, or hemp seeds. All provide better flavor and fun than those fish-oil bullets. This book sets out to help you include them in your diet. After all, where's the decadence in a tablet?

Not just an antidote to depression, the omega-3 fats in herring guard against cognitive decline (what we Irish refer to as our senior moments). No need to agonize over a pesky Rubik's Cube every day. Go boost your brainpower with this laureate-loving recipe instead.

4 pickled herring
  (rollmops will do)
2 hardboiled eggs
1 small red onion
$^1/_2$ apple
Megabunch of flat-leaf parsley
Toast, to serve (try Your New
  Wheat-Free Bread on page 51)

Serves 2-3

With your sharpest knife, finely dice the herring. Repeat with the eggs, onion, and apple. Roughly chop the parsley and tumble everything together. You may want a little yogurt to bring it all together, but this is not considered authentic.

SOLE AND SATAY

Getting teens to eat oily fish can be as easy as stuffing toothpaste back into its tube. That's why we've come up with a satay sauce using nutritious omega oils. They'll get a sneaky dose of omega-3 while tucking into this ridiculously good dish. Shhh.

Chop the baby potatoes in half and steam for 10 minutes.

Meanwhile, finely chop your ginger and crush to a paste with a pestle in a mortar. Mix with the remaining satay ingredients.

As soon as the potatoes are done, spoon the satay sauce over them, and give it all a clumsy stir. The mess is half the charm.

Now is the time to flash-fry each sole fillet. Heat a pan on high. Dot with coconut oil and place each fillet on top. Let the teens do this part—with a bit of luck they'll surprise you one evening in the near future! Lemon sole is delicate, so gently turn after 30 seconds and flash-fry the other side without letting it turn brown. If the pan is not sufficiently hot, the fish may need longer and will brown in the interim. It's a matter of taste I suppose, but I prefer mine snow-white.

Plate up, sprinkle with anything green you may have lurking in the fridge (cilantro? chives? arugula?), and serve with the potato satay. This is *real* fast food, to nourish your body and your creativity.

1 fillet lemon sole per person
Extra virgin coconut oil, to
  flash-fry

For the potato satay:
Enough baby potatoes for 4
1-inch piece of fresh ginger,
  peeled
6-8 tablespoons crunchy
  peanut butter
4 tablespoons Udo's Oil, or
  hempseed or flax oil
3 tablespoons tamari
2 tablespoons mirin
1-2 tablespoons raw honey or
  barley malt extract
1 garlic clove, crushed
Juice of $1/2$ lime

Serves 4

CILANTRO AND POMEGRANATE CEVICHE WITH BOWLS OF FLOPPY FENNEL

xxxxxxxxxxxxxxxxxxxxxxxxxxxxxxxxxxxxxxxxxxxxxxxxxxxxxxxxxxxxxxxxxxxxxxxxxxxxxxxxxxxxxxxxxx

Freshly torn from its plant, cilantro transforms a sad excuse of a salad into a party on a plate. And you're invited.

Unless you have a hotline to Dan Barber's brain, growing cilantro can be a trifle tricky. Best tip? Don't bother with the supermarket plants. They are merely dejected relatives of the real thing and never live longer than their first haircut. Instead, follow these easy steps: (1) Sow salad seeds in a ten-inch deep, well-drained pot. (2) Feed with at least eight hours' sunlight on a windowsill. (3) Keep well watered. (4) Brag to everyone in the office that you GYO and let them rub your halo.

This will feed four, but we double the quantities for supper parties. Very little work involved.

For the floppy fennel:
Juice of 2 limes
1 tablespoon fish sauce
 (nam pla)
1 tablespoon toasted
 sesame oil
2 teaspoons maple syrup
1-2 red onions, finely sliced
 into semicircles
1 fennel bulb, topped and
 tailed and finely sliced

For the ceviche:
1 lb (400 g) super-fresh
 fish like wild sea bass,
 mackerel, or salmon
Juice of 1 blood orange
Juice of 1 lime
2 tablespoons extra virgin
 olive oil
1 tablespoon sea salt flakes
Bunch of fresh cilantro,
 leaves only
Few tablespoons pomegranate
 seeds

Serves 4

To make the floppy fennel, whisk together the lime juice, fish sauce, sesame oil, and maple syrup with a fork. Depending on the size of your limes, you may need to adjust the tartness by adding a smidgeon more sesame oil. Taste. Hover. Leap. Prostrate.

Pour over the thinly sliced red onions and fennel. In a few minutes, the vegetables will turn floppy and sweet, as if inebriated by the dressing. Leave them be and get going on the ceviche.

Ask your fishmonger to skin and bone the fish. If he's really nice, he'll cut them into bite-size pieces for you too. Otherwise, you'll have to see to all three steps yourself before making the ceviche. Tumble the fish with the citrus juice, olive oil, and flakes of salt. Allow to infuse for 1 hour or more in the fridge, but anything past 4 hours will turn the fish rubbery.

Tumble through the torn cilantro and pomegranate seeds. Serve in a large glass bowl and have everyone help themselves alongside the bowls of floppy fennel. Plain quinoa is a great side too with a couple tablespoons of desiccated coconut.

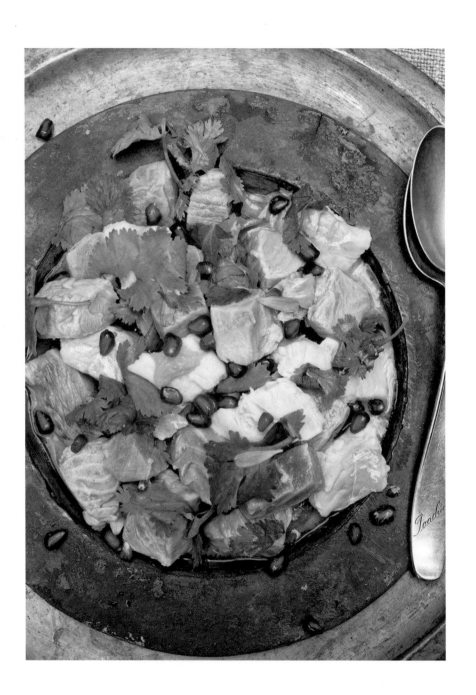

TOMATO AND BANANA BEAN CURRY

xxxxxxxxxxxxxxxxxxxxxxxxxxxxxxxxxxxxxxxxxxxxxxx

A recent study of half a million people confirmed that eating more than 20 grams of processed meat a day was linked to early death. Twenty grams! That's a lick of chorizo. The research covered ten European countries over thirteen years. In other words, it's fairly bulletproof.

This news was announced in the wake of the horsemeat scandal. The clamor of worried shoppers scrambling toward the vegetarian aisles in supermarkets is, frankly, unprecedented. Sales of tofu rocketed by 500 percent.

It's clear that our love affair with sausage sandwiches and shish kebabs has long needed a re-evaluation. It takes up to seven fields of grain to feed one field of cows. No wonder there isn't enough food to feed the world—Daisy's scoffing most of it. With the intensification of global warming and the planet's population ever escalating, never has the case for cutting down on meat been more compelling. But quitting altogether? No thank you.

This is our RDA curry, squeezing loads of nutrient-dense fruit and veggies into one small pot. It's enough for five tummies, freezes well, and also keeps in the fridge for a few days. It's pretty dishy served on a bed of wilted spinach and doesn't require Birkenstocks to enjoy it. Beans are one of the most common foods found in a centenarian's diet, so if you want to live longer and look like vegan superstar Alicia Silverstone, start by taping this recipe to your cupboard door.

1 large onion, diced
2-3 tablespoons extra virgin
    olive oil
Two 14.5 oz (411 g) cans of
    diced tomatoes
One 15 oz (425 g) can of mixed
    beans
5 dried apricots, chopped
2 bananas, sliced
2 tablespoons raisins
2 tablespoons curry powder
Squeeze of lemon juice
2-3 garlic cloves, crushed
Fresh parsley, to garnish
Dollop of natural coconut
    yogurt, to serve
Black pepper, to taste
Sweet brown rice (see page
    141), to serve

Serves 5

Normally the best way to begin a curry is by sweating the onion in olive oil on low heat in a heavy-based saucepan until translucent, but on those seriously swift evenings, just bung it all in together. Add the tomatoes to the onion and bring to a low simmer, at which point you can add the beans, apricots, bananas, raisins, curry powder, and lemon juice. Cook for 15 minutes.

The key to this recipe is to stir through the crushed garlic as soon as the curry is ready, and not before. Divide among 5 plates and drizzle reverently with extra virgin olive oil and torn parsley. Crown with a dollop of live coconut yogurt and maybe a few turns of the black pepper mill and serve with short-grain or sweet brown rice. You will feel your toes sing.

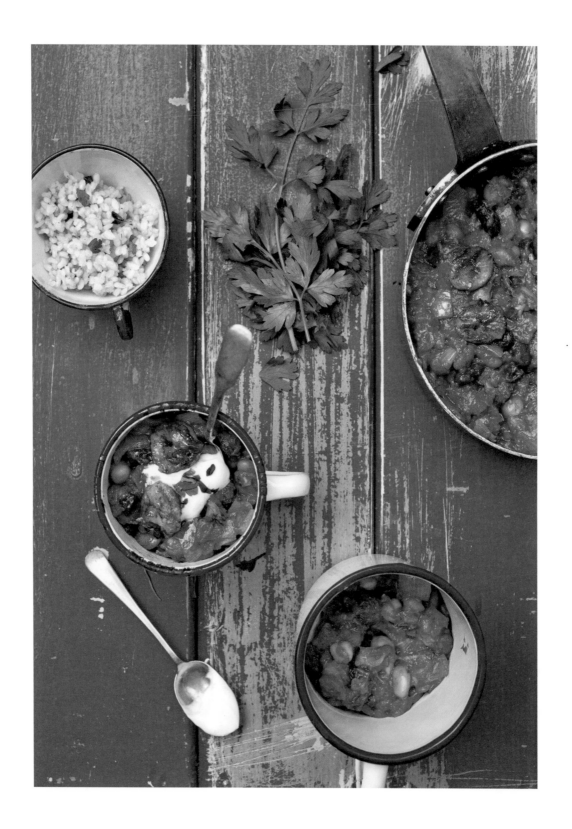

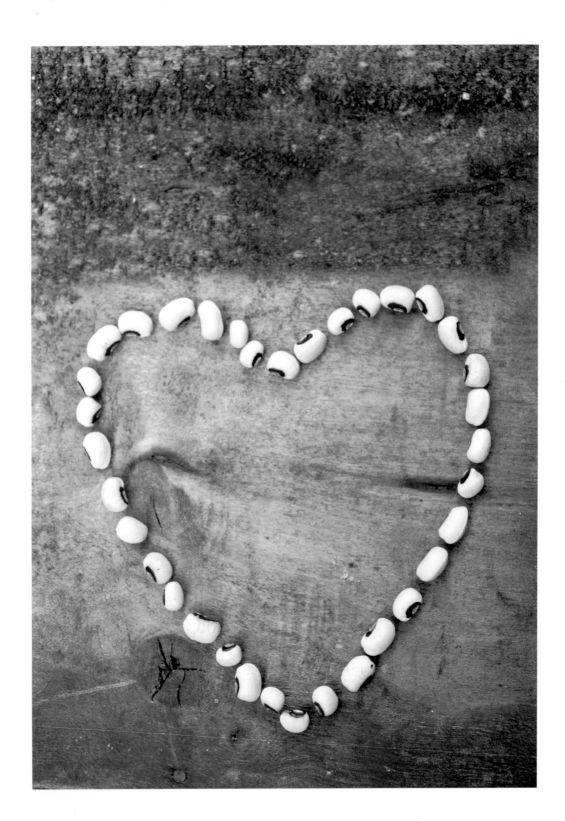

CENTENARIAN'S PINEAPPLE AND GOJI BERRY CURRY
WITH RAITA AND SPINACH

xxxxxxxxxxxxxxxxxxxxxxxxxxxxxxxxxxxxxxxxxxxxxxxxxxxxxxxxxxxxxxxxxxxxxx

Gastroenterologists (the specialists who look after your pipes) recommend eating 30-35 grams of dietary fiber every day. That's because they know that high-fiber diets can lower the risk of developing colon and gastric cancers by 40 percent. One cup of cooked red kidney beans provides 11 grams, while adzuki beans ring in at 17 grams per serving. Want to know the average daily intake? A measly 10 grams. So forget that hideous childhood rhyme and start loving beans. They love you.

There's a secret bonus in this recipe. Pineapple, goji berries, red onions, ginger, garlic, chili, and turmeric are all members of an anti-inflammatory squad. Many are flush with flavonoids too, otherwise known as heavyweight antioxidants that fight aging and disease.

You can play around with the flavors here-try vindaloo, Bengali, or Chinese five spice blend. Let your taste buds vote. No need to stick to canned beans either. We often cook adzuki beans for 20 minutes or butterbeans for 90 minutes before adding them to the tomato base.

Preheat the oven to 350°F (180°C).

The method employed here is more practical than traditional. Tumble the chopped butternut squash or sweet potatoes with a little oil and roast for 40 minutes, until caramelized and soft. You can leave the skin on the squash if it's organic. Quarter the red onions and toss with the chunks of pepper and a splash of oil. Roast on a separate tray from the squash for 20 minutes, until semi-soft. I keep a little raw red onion to mix through the curry before serving. It's up to you.

While the veggies soften in the oven, find your largest casserole dish or stockpot and heat up the canned tomatoes and stock. Add the drained beans, chopped pineapple, goji berries, curry powder, and turmeric. Let this gurgle away for 10-15 minutes, by which time the roasted onions and peppers will be ready.

Remove the tray from the oven and shake the veggies into your pot of spicy tomatoes. Your nostrils should be levitating by now. Turn down the heat very low and prep the last few ingredients while the squash is finishing off in the oven.

(continued)

For the bean curry:
3 cups (450 g) chopped
  butternut squash or sweet
  potato
Splash of extra virgin
  coconut oil
3 red onions
2 red bell peppers, deseeded
  and chopped
Two 14.5 oz (411 g) cans of
  whole tomatoes
1 cup (250 ml) chicken or
  vegetable stock
One 15 oz (425 g) can of mixed
  beans, drained
4 slices of pineapple, skin
  removed and chopped
$1/2$ cup (50 g) dried goji
  berries
2 tablespoons hot curry
  powder
1 teaspoon fresh or ground
  turmeric
2 garlic cloves
1 red chili, deseeded if
  necessary

3-inch piece of fresh ginger,
    peeled
Sea salt flakes

For the spinach:
One and a half 10 oz (284 oz)
    packages of frozen spinach
    for every 2 people
Salt and pepper
Extra virgin olive oil
1 garlic clove, crushed

For the raita:
Cucumber
Mint leaves
Lemon juice
Honey
Natural or coconut yogurt

Serves 8

Crush the garlic, chili, and ginger together with a sprinkle of sea salt flakes in a mortar to make a seriously fragrant paste. These are heroic immune-boosting anti-inflammatory foods. Stir the paste through the curry. The idea is not to cook these ingredient but rather, warm them so their medicinal qualities are not significantly diminished.

Pour 1 inch of boiling water over the spinach and boil for 2 minutes in a small saucepan with a fitted lid. When it's defrosted (no need to murder it), drain very well in a sieve, give it a few turns of the salt and pepper mill, and tickle with olive oil and maybe another lick of garlic.

The raita is a cinch-chop a bit of cucumber and mint. Add a spot of lemon juice and/or honey to natural yogurt, taste, and adjust to your preferences. Spinach and raita are pretty special additions to this meal. Without them, think gin with no tonic.

As soon as the squash is soft, add it to the tomato curry, ramp up the heat and roar at everyone to take their places at the dinner table. Time to plate up.

PUMPKIN FALAFEL

xxxxxxxxxxxxxxxxxxxxxxxx

It's a shame Halloween has monopolized the pumpkin. They're far too fabulous to be dismissed for eleven months of the year.

This vegetable's buttery flesh is stuffed with goodness. There's potassium for hangovers, vitamins A and C to slay superbugs (think Uma Thurman in Kill Bill), and extra carotenoids for those who can't afford to keep up their Botox installments. That's a lot of ammunition for a supposedly ghoulish vegetable.

On the antioxidant radar, pumpkins are almost up there with blueberries and spinach. We like antioxidants because they help prevent the bad LDL cholesterol in our bloodstream from oxidizing. Once oxidation occurs, we're told the likelihood of cholesterol depositing onto blood vessel walls significantly increases. Not sure I like the sound of that.

Heart surgeon Dr. Oz Mehmet has even devised a recipe for pumpkin brownies to entice his clients into eating more of this useful vegetable. According to Dr. Oz, pumpkins are probably one of the best foods we ain't eatin'.

Here's my recipe, based on Allegra McEvedy's (one of my favorite chefs). Deep-frying falafel may taste delish, but isn't recommended for our waistlines or arteries. Shame. More alarmingly, deep-frying food can make your mouth feel like a camel's armpit. Luckily, Allegra designed hers to be baked.

Preheat the oven to 340°F (170°C).

This recipe isn't a science. You're aiming for the falafel to be one-quarter chickpea or chestnut flour. It's really that simple, so use whatever amount of pumpkin you have and adjust the recipe as appropriate.

Roasting pumpkin is a cinch too—no peeling necessary. Just make sure to avoid the monstrous Cinderella ones. Start by cautiously hacking the side of the pumpkin. Chop this flesh into matchbox-size pieces and continue to work your way around the pumpkin. The hardest part is that first slice. Tumble the pieces into a roasting tray with a good splash of coconut or olive oil. Cover with foil. Roast for 45-60 minutes, until sweet and tender. Pumpkin is better overcooked rather than undercooked.

(continued)

1 small field pumpkin, acorn squash, or red kurl squash, cut in pieces and roasted (500 g)

Just over 1 cup (125 g) chickpea flour (aka gram flour) or chestnut flour

2 garlic cloves, crushed

Zest and juice of $^1/_2$ lemon

2-3 tablespoons extra virgin coconut or olive oil

2 tablespoons chopped spring onions

2 teaspoons ground cumin

Black sesame seeds, to garnish

Makes 8-12 falafel

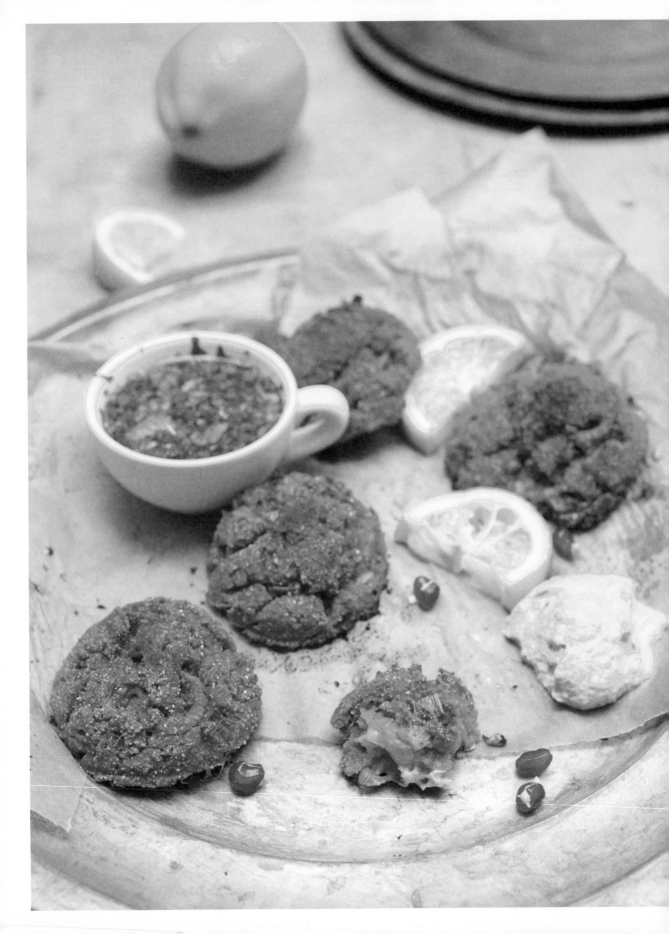

Remove the tray of pumpkin and let the pieces cool completely before handling. If you've roasted more than you need, count yourself lucky. Whiz any leftover pieces with coconut milk, sautéed onions, and a pinch of curry powder to make soup. Or freeze a batch for your next falafel craving.

Raise the oven temperature to 400°F (200°C). Line a baking tray with parchment paper or grease with a lick of olive oil.

Using clean hands, mash together all the falafel ingredients except the black sesame seeds. Put the falafel mix in the freezer for 15-30 minutes to firm up. Mould the chilled mixture into falafels and place on the lined baking tray. I find an ice cream scoop is the best way to shape falafel. If you use teaspoons and patience, you'll double the portions and halve the baking time. Sprinkle with black sesame seeds and cook in the oven for 20-45 minutes, depending on their size.

Try serving alongside thick natural or coconut yogurt, smooth hummus, Maple Mustard Lentils (page 158), or a big bowl of peas. The messier, the better.

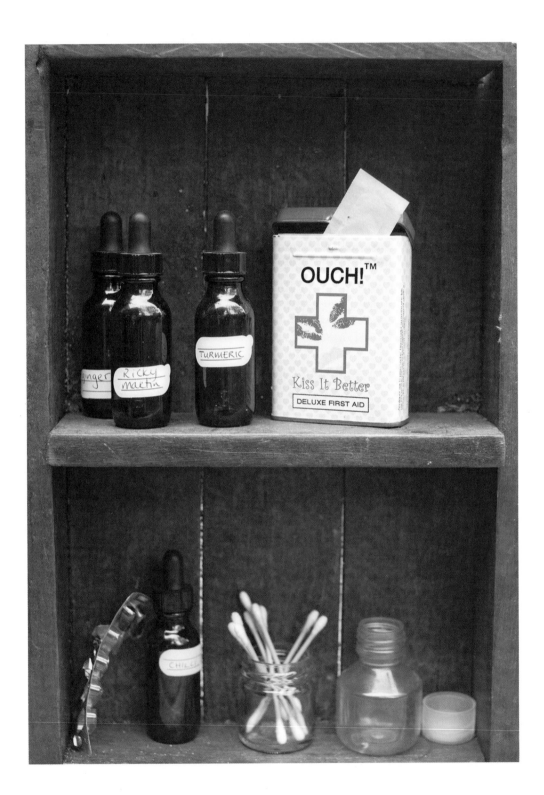

ANTI-INFLAMMATORY ALOO

This famous dish gets its psychedelic glow from poor man's saffron (turmeric). Its high veggie content also helps it feel like a big bowl of sunshine. Anti-inflammatory Aloo isn't the sexiest of names for a Saturday night curry, but did you know that inflammation relates to heaps of common conditions, such as psoriasis, bruising, swelling, hay fever, joint pain, chest infections, IBS, and asthma?

You'll find a hub of ingredients in this aloo to help reduce menacing prostaglandins in the body. There are good prostaglandins and bad prostaglandins. We're told that both manage the inflammatory process. The bad ones morph into inflammatory markers in your bloodstream and can make your body feel like a rusty BMX with a twenty-ton rhino on the Tour de France. Anti-inflammatory foods like turmeric, ginger, goji berries, onions, and chili can help interrupt the life cycle of bad prostaglandins so that less of them end up circulating in your body. Pretty nifty, huh?

Start by peeling and finely chopping the onion and ginger. On the stovetop, heat a heavy-based casserole pot on its lowest setting with a few tablespoons of oil and add your chopped onion, ginger, chili, cumin, mustard seeds, and turmeric. Sweat for 10 minutes. Your nostrils will applaud.

Cut the baby potatoes into generous mouthfuls. Prepare your cauliflower by discarding the outer leaves, breaking into Lego-size florets, and cutting the center stalk into rough cubes. Be sure not to throw this part out—it adds wonderful texture to your aloo. Toss the potatoes, cauliflower, and butter beans with the sautéed onion, coating everything with the spice's golden glow. Pour over the stock and add the goji berries (if using). Bring to a boil, cover with a lid, and let it gurgle for 20-25 minutes, until the veggies are soft but not soggy. They will joyously soak up most of the stock while simmering away. Taste, and season with sea salt and a few turns of the black pepper mill. Serve with fresh cilantro stirred through the gobi.

Other aloo gobi variations include a tablespoon of garam masala, shrimp, peanuts, desiccated coconut, or raw minced garlic stirred through at the end, or a squeeze of lemon just before serving. Let your taste buds vote.

1 large red onion
Thumb-size piece of fresh ginger
Splash of extra virgin coconut or peanut oil
1 green chili, deseeded and finely chopped
1 tablespoon ground cumin
1 tablespoon black mustard seeds (optional)
2 teaspoons ground turmeric
6 baby potatoes
$1/2$ head of cauliflower
1 cup cooked (see page 118) or canned butter beans, drained
2 cups (500 ml) chicken, fish or vegetable stock
$1/4$ cup (25 g) goji berries (optional)
Salt and pepper
Fresh cilantro, to serve

Serves 4

RED DAAL WITH WILTED SPINACH AND A PLUMP POACHED EGG

xxxxxxxxxxxxxxxxxxxxxxxxxxxxxxxxxxxxxxxxxxxxxxxxxxxxxxxxxxxxxxxxxxxxxxx

This dish requires little or no kitchen experience. Unlike beans, red lentils do not need pre-soaking or hours of patience. You'll find most of the ingredients already lurking in your cupboard, making it particularly attractive for unexpected callers.

Research from the British Journal of Pharmacology shows that garlic and ginger contain antibacterial and anti-inflammatory compounds to help soothe anything from swollen tonsils to achy limbs. Did you know most common skin complaints involve inflammation? Dandruff, psoriasis, acne, and eczema–all would benefit from a good frolic with garlic and ginger. Besides, they're outrageously tasty, dead cheap, and will vastly improve a dull date.

1 onion, diced
2 tablespoons extra virgin
  coconut or olive oil
1 cup (190 g) dried red
  lentils, washed
6-8 cloves
2 garlic cloves, finely
  chopped
1 tablespoon mustard seeds
  (whole-grain mustard
  would do)
1 tablespoon minced ginger
1 teaspoon whole black or
  white peppercorns, smashed
Chicken stock or water
3 handfuls of baby spinach
  leaves
3 poached eggs (see page 150)
Nice squeeze of lemon juice
  (optional)

Serves 3

Start by sweating the onion in the oil on a low setting for 10 minutes, until they appear slightly glassy. A heavy-based saucepan is perfect to avoid the onions catching on the bottom of the pan and burning. If you fry the onions at a higher temperature, the oil will chemically change and play with your arteries. It doesn't matter if you use the best cold-pressed extra virgin oil money can buy. High heat, as opposed to gentle warmth, chemically disfigures oil and spoils most of the health benefits it carries. If you suffer from cholesterol or weight problems, it might be worth writing this on the inside of your kitchen cupboard to remind you!

As the onions sweat, in another medium-size saucepan combine the lentils, cloves, garlic, mustard seeds, ginger, and peppercorns. Add enough chicken stock or water to cover the lentils by about $^3/_4$ inches and bring to a boil. Sometimes I do a blend of carrot juice and water to give the lentils a fabulously rich color and sweetness. Adjust the heat so that the lentils putter away rather than violently bubble. Cover and cook for about 12 minutes, then remove from the heat, keep the lid on, and allow to stand on the countertop until tender. Ideally, daal should be saucy, not soupy, so keeping the lid on the pan will naturally steam the lentils for another couple of minutes.

Remove the cloves from the cooked lentils (it helps if you remember exactly how many you popped in) and add the baby spinach and the sautéed onion. Divide among 3 bowls and slip your poached egg on top. Finish off with a generous squeeze of lemon and love.

FLASH-FRIED PLAICE WITH PINK PEPPERCORN SALT AND LEMON DUST

xxxxxxxxxxxxxxxxxxxxxxxxxxxxxxxxxxxxxxxxxxxxxxxxxxxxxxxxxxxxxxxxxxxxxxxxxxxxxxxxxxxxxxxxxxx

That gorgeous Italian Laura Santtini has bewitched me with her Flash Cooking. It's not a diet or a fad. It's a master class in creativity and time poverty. Santtini's mission is to arm your kitchen with an arsenal of explosively tasty spices, finishing salts, and scented yogurts. They are guaranteed to transform your meals, and possibly even your life.

Plaice is a superslim fish that cooks in less than 90 seconds. Not so good from the freezer, so make sure your plaice is hyperfresh. I buy the white-bellied fillets as opposed to the black side because the soft white skin is the best part. Plaice camouflage themselves in the ocean-one side is dark and mottled so that predators above the plaice can't differentiate them from the ocean floor. Their underbelly is white so that predators below them think they are shards of light glistening in the water. Poor things never accounted for crafty fishermen.

Dot of extra virgin coconut
   oil
2 fillets plaice
Zest of 1 small lemon
1 teaspoon pink peppercorns
Pinch of sea salt flakes
Black olives, to serve
Roasted fennel (page 152),
   to serve

Serves 2

Heat a large frying pan on high. When the pan is piping hot, dot with coconut oil and immediately drop the fillets over the oil. Each side should take only 20-40 seconds to cook, during which time you can zest the lemon and crush the pink peppercorns in a mortar. Mix the zest and peppercorns with the flakes of salt and dust each fillet with this finishing touch as soon as you plate up. You'll need to work at a brisk speed.

Plaice is too delicate for lemon juice, so the zest is perfect. A simple bowl of black olives and lightly roasted fennel serves us well.

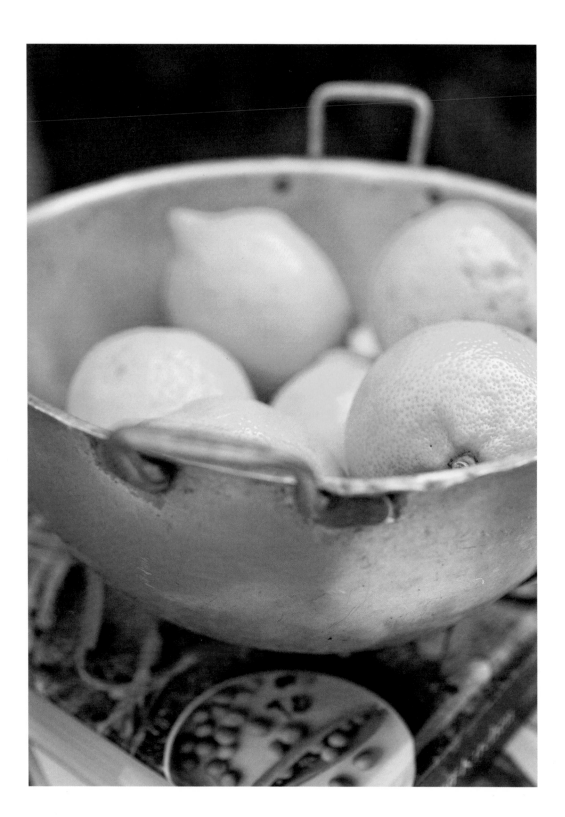

UMAMI BEEF STEW

xxxxxxxxxxxxxxxxxxxxxxxx

Domini Kemp is a badass Irish chef who women want to be and men want to meet. This is her flavor bomb. One of Domini's restaurants, Hatch & Sons Irish Kitchen, pencils it on the menu from time to time. I've seen fans bless themselves in its presence.

Umami is our fifth taste sensation, often underserviced. Scientists refer to this neglected fifth taste bud as the lip-smacking point. Think anchovies, Parmesan cheese, miso, tamari, and prosciutto. Domini uses streaky rashers in the original recipe, but given the fatwa on piggies in our house, we subbed it with umami-rich seaweed and mushrooms.

This freezes really well, so tuck some away for those evenings when you couldn't be bothered to knock up a meal from scratch.

A few good splashes of extra
  virgin olive oil
1¹/₂ lbs (800 g) stewing beef
  or lamb, cut into 1-inch
  chunks
2¹/₂ cups (500 g) wild mixed
  mushrooms (not dried)
2 large onions, chopped
1¹/₂ head of garlic, peeled
  and sliced
Large glass of red wine
Strip of dried wakame or kombu
  (optional)
6 cups (1.5 liters) stock
One 2 oz (55 g) can of
  anchovies
2 heaped tablespoons tomato
  purée
3 bay leaves

For the sweet potato purée:
6 large sweet potatoes
Seasoning

**For the carrot and mango
  purée:**
8 medium carrots, unpeeled
Handful of dried mango
Extra virgin coconut oil

Serves 8

Preheat the oven to 325°F (160°C).

It's quicker to have 2 pans frying simultaneously. Using a heavy-based pan, brown the meat all over in batches. This should take 10–15 minutes. Make sure the meat looks almost caramelized.

Take your biggest ovenproof pot (ideally a cast-iron, heavy-bottomed casserole dish like Le Creuset) and sauté the mushrooms, onions and garlic in small batches in some oil. As they soften and color, transfer to a large plate with the browned meat. Work like this for 15 minutes, until all the beef, mushrooms, and onions are colored and ready to rock. The reason we don't bung them all into one pan is because they will sweat rather than caramelize.

Once the beef has finished browning, deglaze the pan with a large glass of red wine, then transfer to the ovenproof pot. Let the mushrooms, onions, garlic, and kombu or wakame (if using) join the party. Add the stock, anchovies, tomato purée and bay leaves and bring to a simmer.

Pop it into the oven and cook for about 2 hours with a lid on. Turn the heat way down to 250°F (120°C). Cook for another 60 minutes.

To make the sweet potato purée, pop the spuds whole into a hot oven for 1 hour. They will naturally steam in their skins, provided they are not cut or slit. If the potatoes are massive, you'll need an extra 30 minutes' cooking time. Adjust as you feel fit. Sweet potatoes are best when they are really soft, not al dente. Once they are properly cooked, their skins will peel off easily. Mash with tasty seasoning like Herbamare or celery salt. You can purée them in a food processor to achieve a silky-smooth finish. Sweet potatoes behave differently than regular white spuds and can be put through a blender without turning into glue.

For the carrot and mango purée, chop up the carrots and steam with the dried mango for 10–15 minutes. Make sure they are very soft before whizzing in a food processor or a hand-held blender. Add a drop of coconut oil for creaminess.

All 3 dishes can be made 1 or 2 days in advance of a dinner party and reheated when required. In fact, the stew tastes even better when the beef gets a chance to absorb all those umami semiquavers. Amen.

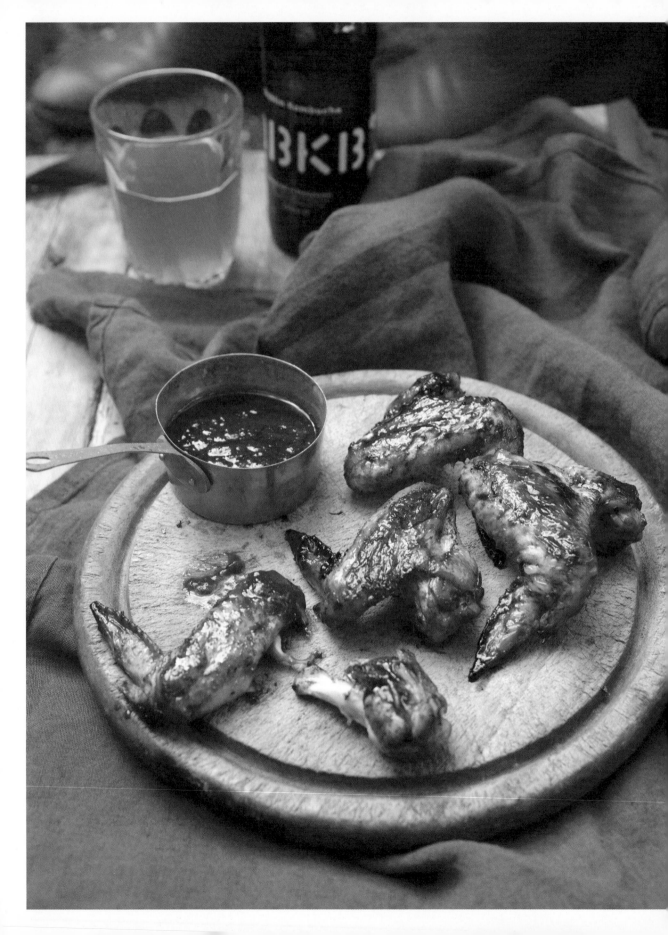

LICKY-STICKY WINGS WITH CHILI SAUCE

xxxxxxxxxxxxxxxxxxxxxxxxxxxxxxxxxxxxxxxxxxxxxxxxxxxxxxxxxxxx

I think cutlery is really odd. Touch is a sense that can heighten taste.
Try this recipe and see for yourself. Serve with your favorite bean sprouts, dressed
with freshly juiced ginger if possible, or a tray of roasted parsnips and carrots.

Preheat the oven to 400°F (200°C).

Carefully remove any stray feathers from the wings
and discard. Throw the wings onto a roasting tray and
drizzle with the lemon juice, honey, oil, and peppercorns. Give everything a jolly good tumble to coat well.
Roast for 40 minutes, shaking the tray whenever you
remember to.

If you are cooking enough wings for 4 people, you will
need 2 trays. The magic in browning wings is to give
them plenty of space and independence on the roasting
tray. The same principle applies to roasting veggies-an
overcrowded tray generates too much steam between the
ingredients, resulting in a soggy, insipid meal.

To make the chili sauce, knock it up with a hand-held
blender or stir together with a fork and strength. The
wings are sufficiently tasty on their own, but the sauce
amps up the reverie. There's something so primal about
chicken wings and great big bowls of licky-sticky yummy.

Around 12 chicken wings
Juice of 1 large lemon
2 tablespoons honey (not
  agave)
2 tablespoons extra virgin
  coconut oil
1 tablespoon black or
  Szechuan peppercorns,
  smashed

For the chili sauce:
2-3 tablespoons barley malt
  extract, raw agave nectar,
  or yacón syrup
2 tablespoons fresh miso
  paste
2 tablespoons cold-pressed
  toasted sesame oil
$^{1}/_{2}$ teaspoon cayenne pepper

Serves 2-3

ROAST CHICKEN WITH IRISH GREMOLATA AND CHARRED PUMPKIN

xxxxxxxxxxxxxxxxxxxxxxxxxxxxxxxxxxxxxxxxxxxxxxxxxxxxxxxxxxxxxxxxxxxxxxxxxxxxxxxxxxxx

Chicken is a special treat in our home, when an occasion demands. We don't think meat is evil. I like Mark Bittman's idea of using meat as a garnish instead of giving meat the lead role. Hugh Fearnley-Whittingstall built on Bittman's idea by publishing a book with vegetables as its entire cast. This may not seem unusual, except that Hugh is Britain's High Priest of Carnivore-ville.

Scientists warn that the amount of meat we eat is unhealthy and unsustainable. Therein lies the problem. If Bittman's resolution seems too darn difficult, another smart option is to buy meat only when it is free range and unprocessed. Meat piracy is a curse.

1 large organic, free-range, or higher-welfare chicken
1 large fennel bulb (optional)
1 large, juicy lemon
2 tablespoons extra virgin coconut oil
Sea salt flakes

For the Irish gremolata:
Pinch of sea veggies (arame is excellent)
4 garlic cloves
Zest and juice of 2 lemons
1 cup extra virgin olive oil
1 cup (50 g) parsley, roughly chopped

For the charred pumpkin:
1 small organic pumpkin
Extra virgin coconut or olive oil

Serves 6

Take your chicken out of the fridge 40 minutes before cooking. It's also a good idea to clear the kitchen sink so that when you wash your hands after touching the bird, you don't transfer bacteria to your dishes.

Preheat the oven to 450°F (230°C). Quarter the fennel (if using) and place in the center of a roasting tray. Carefully remove the chicken's packaging and gently place the bird on top of the fennel. Wash your hands thoroughly after handling the bird, especially if you have children dancing at your heels.

Roll the lemon under the palm of your hand (a microwave will briefly warm it up to get the juices spilling). Halve the lemon and rub the bird all over with it. Squeeze the juice into the tray and pop the empty lemon halves in the bird's cavity. Dot with the coconut oil and season with a flurry of salt flakes.

Place the tray in the oven and turn it down to 400°F (200°C). Cook a 3$\frac{1}{2}$-pound bird for approximately 1 hour 20 minutes. The top of the chicken leg bones will look dry and prominent once the bird is cooked and the meat should easily come away from the bone. If not, leave in the oven for longer.

Meanwhile, to make the Irish gremolata, soak the arame in water for 10 minutes to rehydrate. If you've chosen a different sea veggie, follow the instructions on the packet. Discard the soaking water once it's ready and roughly chop. Use a kitchen grater to mince each clove of garlic. Follow with the lemon zest. Squeeze the juice from both lemons and add the oil. Add the parsley and give it all a good shake in a jam jar. Set aside.

Slice the pumpkin into wedges using vigor and vigilance. Scoop out its stringy nest and dice the flesh into matchbox-size pieces. If it's organic, keep the skin on—saves on time and gives extra nutrition. I've also noticed that organic pumpkins are 10 times tastier than conventional ones. Tumble the pumpkin pieces onto a large baking tray and give it a good lick of coconut or olive oil. Roast on high for 45-65 minutes, or until it starts browning and caramelizing around the edges. The same temperature as the chicken is fine. Shake the tray once or twice during roasting to share the juices around the pan and let your nostrils party.

The pumpkin can start cooking 1 hour before the chicken finishes cooking so that it all comes out of the oven at the same time. While the chicken rests, you can switch off the oven, leave the door ajar, and keep the pumpkin and guests warm.

If you have time, roast a tray of carrots too or prepare the carrot and mango purée on page 192. This will help stretch the meal to 8 and bump up your veggie intake.

10-HOUR SHOULDER OF LAMB WITH CRUSHED CHICKPEAS AND THE BEST SAUCE YOU'RE EVER LIKELY TO TASTE

xxxxxxxxxxxxxxxxxxxxxxxxxxxxxxxxxxxxxxxxxxxxxxxxxxxxxxxxxxxxxxxxxx

Here's some slow-cooked lamb that effortlessly falls off the bone. Let it cozy up to some messy chickpea smash and a scorching hot Middle Eastern mojo. This recipe was designed to help mend marriages.

For the slow-cooked lamb:
1 shoulder of mutton
  (an older lamb)
2 tablespoons balsamic
  vinegar
Few tablespoons sumac
  (optional)

For the crushed chickpeas:
2¹/₂ cups (500 g) dried
  chickpeas
1 teaspoon bicarbonate of
  soda
1 strip of kombu seaweed
  (optional)
¹/₂ cup (140 g) cashew butter
3 garlic cloves, crushed
3 tablespoons tamari (or
  generous seasoning)
Squeeze of lemon juice

For the hot anchovy mojo:
One 2 oz (55 g) can of
  anchovies (8-10 anchovies)
3-5 mixed medium chilies,
  deseeded
3 garlic cloves, crushed
1 red bell pepper, finely
  chopped
1 yellow bell pepper, finely
  chopped
2 large bunches of fresh
  cilantro
1 tablespoon ground cumin
1 tablespoon dried oregano
Juice of 1 lemon

Start tonight by soaking the chickpeas in cold water. Tomorrow, drain and discard the soaking water. Tip the chickpeas into your largest heavy-based pan with the bicarb and ramp up the heat. Stir for 30 seconds without burning the bum off the pan. Pour in 2-3 liters of water and the strip of kombu seaweed (if using). Bring to a rolling boil and cook for 1 hour. While you want the chickpeas to be soft and cooked, try not to let them go mushy. Taste a chickpea every so often and decide how soft you like them to be. A good test is to press one between your middle finger and thumb-the chickpea should just about submit to pressure.

Remove from the heat, drain, and set three-quarters of the chickpeas aside. Blitz the other one-quarter in a food processor with the cashew butter and garlic. Add a few good splashes of ice-cold water from the fridge, just to loosen it up. Finish whizzing to a smooth cream.

Roll the cream into the drained chickpeas and gently crush some of the chickpeas to let in the flavors of the smooth sauce. Douse with enough tamari and lemon juice to suit your fancy. You can leave this big pot of crushed chickpeas covered in a warm oven until required.

To make the hot anchovy mojo, give all the ingredients a jolly good whiz in your food processor, but not with a hand-held blender. Food processors give chunkier textures, whereas hand blenders are basically creamers. As spicy, captivating, and sparkling as that first kiss, this sauce is high octane.

To cook the lamb, preheat the oven to 425°F (220°C).

Rub the lamb with the balsamic vinegar and sumac (if using) and place on a roasting pan with high edges. Bring to room temperature before blasting at high heat in the oven for 20 minutes. Turn down the heat to 275°F (140°C) and cook for 8 hours.

Pull some meat away from the bone after 6-8 hours to check how it's doing. If you are doubling up to feed 10, then make sure to give the lamb a few extra hours. Increasing the quantity of food in the oven often dilutes the heat and can result in undercooking, especially at this temperature. Similarly, if the lamb is a small spring shoulder, it probably needs only 6 hours and will feed fewer people. The meat is done as soon as it falls from the bone and practically dissolves in your mouth.

We find the best way to serve this is by piling every-thing on the table. A simple crisp salad dressed in lemon juice and black pepper can help stretch out the number of mouths to feed.

Dash of sherry vinegar
  (to taste)
Great big glug (120 ml) of
  extra virgin olive oil

Serves 5

CHOCOLATE CHILI CON CARNE WITH COCONUT YOGURT

xxxxxxxxxxxxxxxxxxxxxxxxxxxxxxxxxxxxxxxxxxxxxxxxxxxxxxxxxxxxxxxxxxxxxx

If you are a feral carnivore, like my husband, here's a good way of introducing more beans and veggies to your diet without feeling oppressed. The overtones are there (what man won't wolf down a chili con beast?), but so is the nutritional purchase. It doesn't actually taste of chocolate, but rather, utilises cacao powder as another spice in the mix.

By downloading some good podcasts at RadioLab.org, you'll prep this before you even realize it. Put your feet up and enjoy the dance your nostrils will do over the next 2 hours. Serve with great big dollops of cultured coconut yogurt, macerated red onions, and exceptional company.

1½ cups (270 g) dried kidney
  beans, soaked overnight
2 onions
2 red bell peppers
1 large carrot
4 garlic cloves
Extra virgin olive or coconut
  oil, for sautéing
2 tablespoons tomato purée
  (optional)
1 tablespoon dried oregano
1 tablespoon raw cacao powder
1 tablespoon sweet or hot
  paprika (optional)
1 cinnamon stick
Good pinch of dried chili
  flakes
Large pinch of coconut sugar
1 lb (500 g) minced beef
One 28 oz (794 g) can diced
  tomatoes
Just over 2 cups (300 ml)
  vegetable or beef stock
Salt and pepper
1 tablespoon ground cumin
2-4 squares dark or raw
  chocolate (optional)

First off, soak the dried kidney beans overnight. The next day, prep the veggies. I find the easiest way to dice the onions is to cut each onion in half, from root to toe. Peel and place the flat part on the chopping board. With a slicing action, make little matchsticks from the onion lengthwise, but not quite cutting all the way to the root end so that they are still held together. Now slice across the matchsticks.

Roughly chop the bell peppers and carrot into bite-size chunks, discarding the seeds and stalks. Slice your garlic and line up all your dried spices and herbs. Now you're ready to cook.

Heat a little oil in your largest sauté pan or frying pan (I have 2 going at the same time to speed things up). Sweat the onions first, stirring regularly for 10 minutes, until they become glassy. Put them aside, then sauté the peppers and carrot until soft but not browned. Add the garlic toward the end, along with the tomato purée, spices, and coconut sugar (if using). Cook for a good 5 minutes and let your nostrils samba. Remove from the heat and pile on top of the resting onions.

Now whack up the heat and brown the beef all over. It needs to be browned or the end result will be disappointingly insipid. You may need to do this in 2 batches.

Tip in the soaked kidney beans (canned is OK in an emergency), canned tomatoes, and stock. Don't worry

(continued)

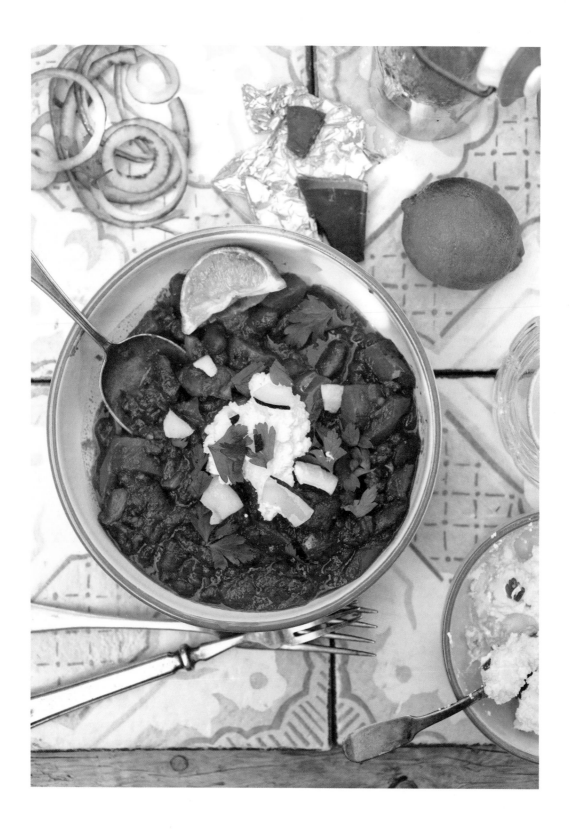

To serve:
1 small red onion
1 really juicy lime
1 tablespoon fish sauce
  (nam pla)(optional)
Fistful of fresh cilantro
  (optional)
Natural coconut yogurt

Serves 10-12

if it looks a little icky. The pot will transform in a few hours. Stir in the veggies, pop a lid on, and let it paddle on a low heat for 2-3 hours. It's done as soon as the beans are soft but not mushy.

Taste, tickle with salt and pepper, and add the cumin and dark chocolate to liven it up. If you feel it needs more pungency, add some yeast extract, blackstrap molasses, or chopped anchovies. Sometimes I do, sometimes I don't.

To serve, cut the red onion in half and finely slice into semicircles. Squeeze the lime over the onions and allow them to party with the fish sauce. Top each bowl of chili con carne with a little macerated red onion, fresh cilantro (if using), and a great big dollop of cultured coconut yogurt in place of sour cream. It's the holy trinity to a good con carne.

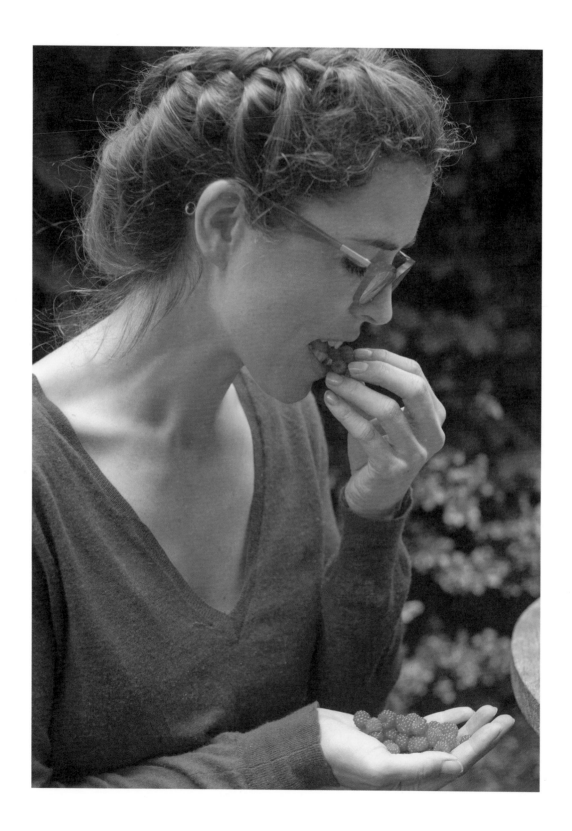

Tasty Healthy Treats

I'm through with guilt.

Looking back, I could never get enough sugar hits. I was an addict.
Everything I did related to or led to my next sugar fix.
I even convinced myself that college projects required
gallons of coffee and jelly beans to charge my brain cells.
I couldn't possibly perform without them.

Sound familiar?

Having to give up junk food was like a bad break-up with the
love of my life. Sudden. Undesired. Unexpected. Grief smothered my
senses like a diaphanous veil over my entire body. I struggled deeply
to wave good-bye to the things I loved in life: my chocolate bars,
ice cream, cupcakes, panna cotta. Clearly, they did not love me back.
Like all cases of unrequited love, I had to get over myself,
move on, or drown in a pool of self-pity.

Here were my choices: Ignore the medical advice I was given
and dig my way to the grave with my teeth? Or nosedive into an apron
and role-play with Anthony Bourdain?

I chose the latter.

Today, my body is in balance. There are no sugar binges or episodes
of overeating. That's because my cravings are satisfied with real
food that nourishes my neurotransmitters in a way
that white sugar and flour never could.

It's *sooo* good to leave the wheat-sugar-dairy circus, to let your
body samba to something less generic and more wholesome. Do it!
If you feed your body, your body will feed you. So here are
loads of treats to help turn your naughty cravings into a
nutritional hit. A word of caution: your wings will go wild and
your toes may take off. *Sláinte!*

**Psst. . . page 12 has a whole lot more information about all
the sweet alternatives available to you.**

Raw Cacao Nib Toffee ------------

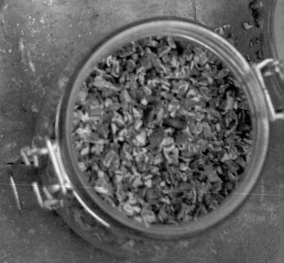

------------ Goji Berry Halva

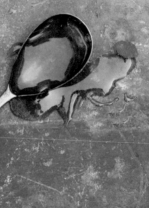

GOJI BERRY HALVA

>>>>>>>>>>>>>>>>>>>>>>>>

This is like a smoochy fudge. It's quite possibly my favorite recipe.

We know that good bone health is intimately linked to what we eat. Dr. Marilyn Glenville, specialist in women's health, is dubious about dairy's monopoly on calcium in our diet. Why, Glenville asks, is our rate of osteoporosis much higher than Japan's, where they don't even eat dairy? A good question. Glenville is not alone. New York Times best-selling author Dr. Joel Fuhrman doesn't rate dairy at all. Fuhrman's medical research and experience as a GP have entirely reversed his thinking about dairy. Worthy of further head-scratching.

So let's explore alternative sources to dairy without having to mourn our cheese board. These include canned salmon and sardines, barley grass, chickpeas, broccoli, figs, sesame seeds, tahini, almonds, hazelnuts, and green leafy vegetables. This Goji Berry Halva is a great place to start.

Melt the coconut oil on very gentle heat. Stir in the maple syrup, vanilla, and salt. Continue to heat for 2 minutes.

With a fork, beat through the tahini, goji berries, and hemp seeds (if you don't have hemp seeds, no worries). Keep some gojies to tickle the top. Scrape half the mixture into a small rectangular container lined with cling wrap. Dribble runny honey over it and scrape the remaining mixture on top of the honey. Prod it with a fork and give it a swirl to move the honey about without incorporating it into the tahini. Think caramel swirls.

Freeze for 4 hours. Just like ice cream, it must be stored in the freezer or else it will melt into a holy mess. Slice big wedges from it and marvel at its virtuous decadence.

3 tablespoons extra virgin coconut oil

Up to $1/2$ cup (125 ml) maple or brown rice syrup

1 teaspoon vanilla extract or powder

1 teaspoon sea salt flakes

$1^1/_4$ cups light tahini

4 tablespoons goji berries

2 tablespoons hemp seeds (optional nutritional boost)

2-3 tablespoons runny raw honey

Makes 30 servings

RAW CACAO NIB TOFFEE

>>>>>>>>>>>>>>>>>>>>>>>>>>>>>>

Apparently, women think about chocolate more then men. Some scientists think this is because eating cacao helps release a cavalry of dopamine in the female brain, the same substance released during orgasm. It's even been suggested that when women eat raw chocolate, it affects activity in the cerebral hemisphere responsible for regulating sexual desire. Only one way to find out. . .

$^1/_2$ cup (125 ml) date syrup
3 tablespoons extra virgin
  coconut oil
1$^1/_4$ cups light tahini
3 tablespoons raw cacao nibs
2 tablespoons carob powder
2 teaspoons vanilla extract
Pinch of sea salt flakes

Makes 25-30 servings

Melt the date syrup and coconut oil together over low heat. Add the remaining ingredients, mushing with a fork. Ensure the oil is well mixed. Taste, and adjust with vanilla or sweetener. Work quickly, as the oil will begin to separate from the other ingredients as soon as it starts cooling. It needs a warm environment.

Line a small rectangular container (a little lunchbox perhaps?) with cling wrap so that it comes out over the sides. Transfer your gorgeous gooey gloss into the lined container and tickle with more cacao nibs (if you have any left).

Transfer to the freezer for 4 hours before indulging. Store it there too, as it melts quite quickly at room temperature.

FANCY PANTS LÚCUMA FUDGE

>>>>>>>>>>>>>>>>>>>>>>>>>>>>>>>>>>>

I'm a firm believer in the idea that healthy eating should never tax your taste buds. This recipe has an authentic fudgy feel, but with none of the wicked additives or cosmetic gunk. It practically levitates with goodness.

Ever look twenty years older on a Sunday morning? Or sport a dirty big hangover? This recipe will help. Lúcuma is a fancy pants fruit from South America, good enough for the gods and maybe even for Satan. Its creamy flesh falls between an avocado and an egg yolk-a killer combo. Its perfume will drive your senses wild.

Line a very small container with cling wrap. Gently melt the coconut oil over low heat and stir in the remaining ingredients with a fork. If you intend to use a vanilla pod, split it along the side lengthwise, carefully peel the pod open, and using the blade of a knife, scoop out its fabulous black seeds. Add to the fudge mix, which should look like wet sand by now. Taste, and adjust the sweetness or saltiness to your preferences.

Spoon into your lined container and let it set in the fridge before cutting into chunks of fudge. It should be ready to devour in 1 hour.

4 tablespoons extra virgin coconut oil
8 tablespoons ground almonds
3 tablespoons lúcuma powder
2 tablespoons maple syrup or raw honey
1 vanilla pod (optional) or 1 teaspoon vanilla extract
Sprinkle of decent unrefined salt, like Himalayan pink rock salt

Makes 12 servings

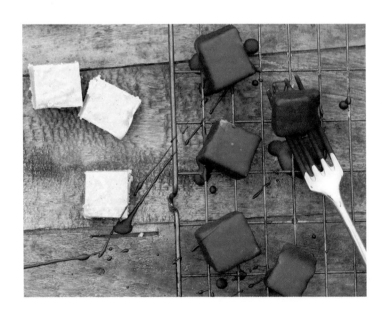

LEMON WHOOPIE PIES

>>>>>>>>>>>>>>>>>>>>>>>>>

Whoopie pies are teeny custard cream cakes with a personality all their own. Every time my son confides that these whoopie pies are his "favorite burgers in the world," my chest swells. I think he's an aspiring vegetarian. Or con artist. It's so hard to tell at three, but the pride is definitely undisputed and comical in equal measure.

When I'm baking for kiddies' birthday parties, I use organic cream cheese instead for the vanilla custard cream. If any of their buddies are lactose intolerant, the filling below does the trick.

For the whoopie pies:
$^1/_2$ cup (65 g) coconut flour
$^1/_2$ cup (50 g) ground almonds
Zest of 1 small lemon
2 tablespoons desiccated
  coconut
2 teaspoons baking powder
$^1/_2$ teaspoon ground turmeric
$^1/_2$ teaspoon sea salt
4 medium eggs
$^1/_2$ cup (125 ml) extra virgin
  coconut oil
$^1/_2$ cup (125 ml) runny honey or
  brown rice syrup (not maple)
Good squeeze of lemon juice

For the vanilla custard
  cream:
1 cup (150 g) cashews, soaked
  in water overnight
$^1/_2$ cup (125 ml) water
$^1/_4$ cup (60 ml) raw agave
  nectar, barley malt
  extract, or brown rice
  syrup (not maple)
2 teaspoons vanilla extract
  or powder
Squeeze of lemon juice
  (optional kick)
$^1/_2$ cup (125 ml) extra virgin
  coconut oil, melted

Makes 10 large or 20 small
  pies

Preheat the oven to 340°F (170°C). Line 2 trays with parchment paper.

To make the cookie base, you'll be using 2 separate bowls. In the first bowl, stir together the dry ingredients. The second bowl wants the wet ingredients (eggs, oil, natural syrup, and lemon juice).

Add the dry ingredients to the wet and mix well. Spoon little puddles onto the lined baking trays. You may need to cook the whoopies in batches, especially if they're teeny tiny ones. Bake large whoopies for 15–18 minutes. If you made smaller whoopies, they'll require only 12–15 minutes.

Remove from the oven and allow to set for 15 minutes before transferring them from their tray and sandwiching with the vanilla custard cream.

To make the vanilla custard cream, discard the soaking water from the cashews. Blitz the nuts in a high-speed food processor with the fresh water, natural syrup, vanilla, and optional lemon for a good 2 minutes.

Meanwhile, gently melt the solid coconut oil until liquid. While the motor is still running, slowly add the coconut oil to the whizzed cashews (like you would if making mayonnaise). Blitz until smooth rather than grainy. The custard cream tends to thicken once chilled for a few hours, so don't panic if it looks like milk.

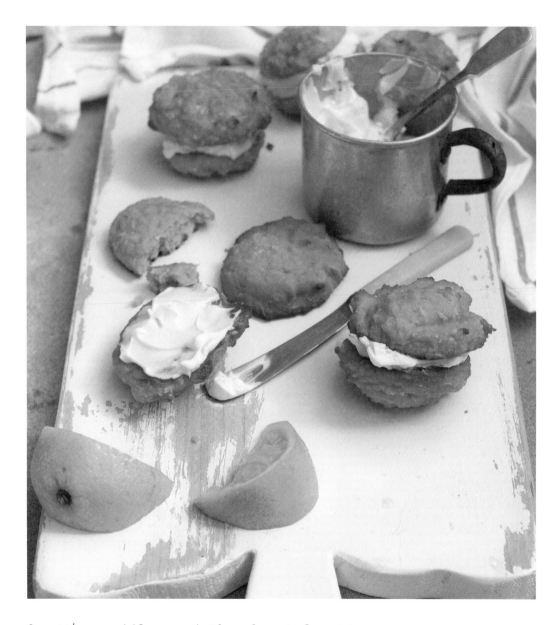

Once it's spreadable, use a knife or fancy implement to slather the filling over a whoopie base, then top with another cookie. The custard cream should be chilled enough to stay firmly in place and hold the whoopie pie together. Take a deep breath, put on some Frank Sinatra, and nosedive into the largest one.

DELINQUENT BROWNIES

These brownies will fool the most ardent of brownie bingers. Not as saccharine as regular cane sugar, coconut blossom sugar offers a burnt toffee kick to everything it caresses. It's not heavily processed either. The sap of the coconut flower is dehydrated to form honeyed crystals. While coconut sugar can be classified as a palm sugar, it is not to be confused with regular palm sugar, which is no friend to the diabetic. Coconut sugar is thought to have a low glycemic value-good news for hyperactive children, diabetics, and bored sedentary workers.

I've used goat's butter in response to many requests over the years to include it in my online recipe portal. This won't suit everyone, but it can be a great alternative for those who react to cow's milk, like my mother. Goat's milk and goat's butter appear to be more alkaline than cow's milk, appealing to those on a calcium-retention diet or alkalizing menus.

The ingredients for these brownies need to be measured in grams. For more on this, see page 8. Don't panic-it's just a fling.

2 large bars (250 g) 85% dark
    chocolate
7 oz (200 g) goat's butter
1 cup (100 g) ground almonds
    or almond flour
2 teaspoons baking powder
4 medium eggs
1¹/₃ cups (250 g) coconut
    blossom sugar

Makes 16-20

Preheat the oven to 350°F (180°C). Line a 9 x 13 inch baking tray with parchment paper and set aside.

Slowly melt most of the chocolate (keep back 30-40 grams) with the goat's butter over a bain-marie. All this means is a saucepan of ³/₄ inches of water simmering away and a shallow bowl fit snugly on top in place of a lid. This is where you'll melt the butter and choccie. If the bowl gets too hot the chocolate will go lumpy, so take it off the heat as soon as you see the ingredients melding. Sometimes the water can turn from a mannerly simmer to a violent boil when you're not watching.

Chop the remaining chocolate into mini chunks, throw into a separate bowl, and stir through the ground almonds and baking powder.

In a very large bowl, beat together the eggs and sugar with an electric whisk until creamy. The mixture will aerate and change color slightly, so don't be overly alarmed. Fold in the ground almond mix and the melted chocolate. Swiftly transfer to your prepared dish with a spatula, before all the lovely air bubbles pop.

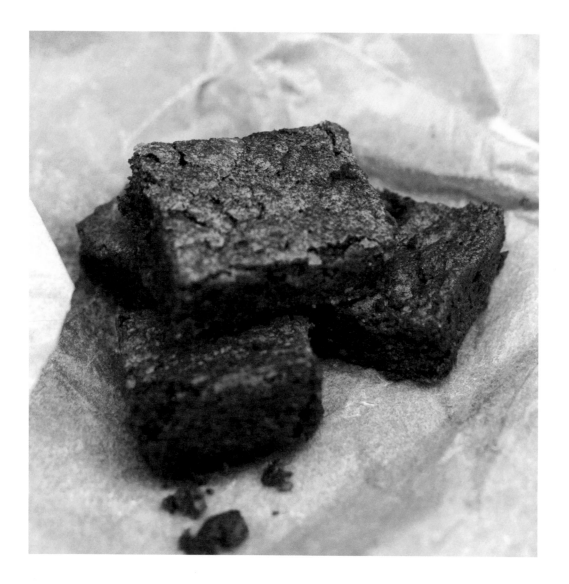

Bake for 30-35 minutes. Use the chocolate bowl and
sticky spatula as currency with your kids-after all,
there's washing up to be done and tired feet to be
massaged.

Once the brownies are cooked, remove and let them cool
overnight in a locked room. Brownies improve exponen-
tially in the fridge, so try to resist looting the tray
until they've sufficiently chilled.

DARK PEANUT BUTTER BROWNIES

>>

Chocolate is a vaccine against bad moods. Something explosive happens in my veins as well as my mouth. According to scientists, this is because of a neurochemical called dopamine. Once stirred, dopamine can initiate an electrical cavalry through the veins and hit every imaginable spot. And I mean every spot. High levels of dopamine are associated with increased motivation, neuroaerobics, and general rí rá agus ruaile buaile-all diplomatic speak for better nookie.

Luckily for us, Mother Nature gave the cacao bean lots of heart-healthy flavanols and magnesium. Both nutrients are loyal friends of the cardiovascular system, helping blood flow and circulation. In fact, I believe the smell of chocolate can send a feline's pulse into a frenzy. Quite the defibrillator.

This endorsement of chocolate comes with a rather large qualification: it must be raw or dark. Untreated, raw cacao is the nutritional heavyweight champion of chocolate. Next best is 85% dark chocolate-indecently rich and muscular. Anything else is disqualified, especially the white or milk varieties. Now for some irritating infor- mation: caffeine (in coffee or chocolate) prompts the body to release stored sugars in our system. This is bad news for diabetics or candida warriors. Caffeine's physi- ological effect can be just as pernicious as sugar. Too much, and we're in trouble.

The ingredients for these brownies are best measured in grams. For more on this, see page 8.

4 tablespoons crunchy peanut
 butter
1-2 tablespoons maple syrup
1 large bar (125 g) 85% dark
 chocolate
3^1/$_2$ oz (100 g) goat's butter
 (see note on page 212)
2 medium eggs
1 cup (125 g) rapadura sugar
 or coconut blossom sugar
^{1}/$_2$ cup ground almonds, almond
 flour, hemp protein powder,
 or gluten-free plain flour
1 teaspoon gluten-free
 baking powder

Makes 10-12

Preheat the oven to 350°F (180°C). Line a small square baking pan (8 x 8 inches) with parchment paper.

Beat the peanut butter and maple syrup together in a cup using a fork and litter the lined baking pan with baby blobs. Set aside.

Slowly melt the chocolate with the goat's butter over a bain-marie. All this means is a saucepan of ^{3}/$_4$ inches of water simmering away and a shallow bowl fit snugly on top in place of a lid. This is where you'll melt the butter and choccie. If the bowl gets too hot the chocolate will go lumpy, so take it off the heat as soon as you see some action.

In a very large bowl, beat together the eggs and sugar with an electric whisk until creamy. Stir through the flour or hemp and the baking powder, then fold in the melted chocolate. Swiftly transfer to your prepared pan with a spatula. Bake for approximately 18 minutes.

Once the brownies are cooked, remove and let them cool overnight in a locked room. Store in the fridge or other chilled hiding place.

ITALIAN AND RICH

>>>>>>>>>>>>>>>>>>>>>>>>

Make David Blaine proud-turn your cravings into a nutritional hit by using avocado in place of cream, and prunes in place of sugar. If you're leery about using them, don't be. Their flavor is muted by the cacao content. This Gianduja-style torte is so darn scrumptious, it feels illicit.

For the base:
6-8 soft prunes or soaked dates
1 cup (135 g) roasted hazelnuts
1/4 cup (25 g) cocoa or cacao powder
1/4 cup (60 ml) maple or date syrup
Handful of walnuts or pecans
2 tablespoons ground flaxseeds

For the ganache topping:
2 Medjool dates, pre-soaked
1 large avocado, stone and skin removed
1/2 cup (50 g) cacao or cocoa powder
1/4 cup (60 ml) maple or date syrup (not honey)
2 tablespoons hazelnut butter
1 teaspoon tamari
1 teaspoon vanilla extract

Serves 14

To make the base, add the listed ingredients to your food processor and pulse until it starts to stick together. You're looking for a clumpy nut texture, not a purée. Make sure your prunes or dates are plump and juicy, otherwise the mixture won't behave. Soak them in a spot of water for 10 minutes before using if you think this will help.

Once pulsed, scrape the base mixture into a pre-lined pan, one that's about half the size of a magazine page. Refrigerate straightaway-I find the base easier to manipulate into place later, when it's chilled.

Now get going on your filling. Whiz all the filling ingredients together with a hand-held blender or food processor. Process until lusciously smooth. Taste to see if it reaches your serotonin and dimples. If not, adjust accordingly: more maple to sweeten, more tamari for depth, more cacao for richness. Set aside.

As soon as the base is cold, press firmly down with the back of a spoon or your fingertips. Fold the filling on top and set for 4 hours in the fridge. Provided it remains in the fridge, it should last for up to 6 days. Pending diligence and discipline, of course.

SEA SALT PROBIOTIC CHOCOLATES

>>>

Probiotic means pro-life. Naturally fermented food like yogurt is brimming with live probiotic bacteria to keep your internal ecosystem in balance. I understand how foul this may sound, but trust me, these guys are on our side. Without healthy strains of live bacteria, our food would not be sufficiently broken down in our guts or absorbed by our bodies. Thrush, bloating, and dodgy bowel movements tend to be the most common symptoms of intestinal imbalance.

If you can't have natural yogurt, look for alternative sources of probiotics in fermented foods such as sauerkraut, kimchi, unpasteurized miso, and coconut yogurt. Or these chocolates. We use them as currency in our house when necessary. Our toddlers will sing Humpty Dumpty in Mandarin for them. So will my husband.

Melt the cacao butter in a bain marie. All this means is placing the broken shards of butter in a shallow bowl set over a pan of barely simmering water. Make sure the bowl is at least 10cm above the simmering water. Remove from the heat and let the cacao butter naturally melt over the hot water for 5 minutes.

Blitz the remaining ingredients (except the raw cacao powder for dusting) in a food processor. Keep the motor running and slowly add the melted cacao butter in a steady stream. The addition of $^1/_4$ teaspoon cayenne pepper is rumoured to make your tongue dance and your pulse quicken. Just saying.

Refrigerate in the same bowl, with the blade intact, for about 1–3 hours. If the mixture seems too hard or you've forgotten about it in the fridge, blitz it again to loosen it up. (That's why it's useful to leave the blade in.)

Put the raw cacao powder in a bowl or shallow plate. Roll the mixture into little bonbons between your palms, then drop into the raw cacao powder. They can be frozen for up to 3 months. Glory be to the icebox!

$^1/_4$ (65 ml) melted cacao butter
$^1/_2$ cup (125 ml) raw agave, barley malt extract or brown rice syrup
$^1/_3$ cup (35 g) cacao or cocoa powder
$^1/_4$ cup (70 g) cashew butter
2 tablespoons hot water
2 tablespoons hazelnut butter (or more cashew butter)
1 tablespoon probiotic powder
1 teaspoon vanilla extract or powder
$^1/_2$ teaspoon flaky sea salt
3 tablespoons raw cacao powder, to dust

Makes 40-50

BEETROOT CANDY

>>>>>>>>>>>>>>>>>>

Tiny titans of flavor, no one would guess these candies are scrupulously healthy. Underneath their neon pink dusting lies some of Mother N's finest superfoods: beetroot, seaweed, and raw almonds.

That bold pigment that gives beetroot its Harry Potter glimmer is where the magic lies. Deep red-colored foods like beetroot and onions store powerful chemicals called betacyanins. These compounds love your liver and are believed to support the body's detoxification process. This might be why beets have charmed every detox clinic from North America to the West of Ireland.

You don't need to stick to beetroot powder for the recipe to work-try a Peruvian powdered fruit called lúcuma. Apparently lúcuma is the maple syrup of South America. A mere whiff of this ambrosial substance has the ability to drive the feminine persuasion wild. Move over, Justin Bieber, there's a new fixation on the block.

15 plump Medjool dates
2 tablespoons almond or
  cashew butter
2 tablespoons extra virgin
  coconut oil
1 tablespoon spirulina
1 teaspoon tamari
2 tablespoons beetroot
  powder, to dust

Makes 30-35 candies

Destone the dates before dropping them into a food processor. Add the remaining ingredients except the beetroot powder. Whiz on a low speed for 1-2 minutes.

Using a teaspoon amount, mold the candy mix into teeny bonbons. Your hands will become slippery, aiding the process. Expect to get around 30-35 candies from the batch, depending on how many times the teaspoon falls into your mouth.

Chill for 24 hours before rolling in the beetroot powder. Any sooner, and the candy will drink up the coating. No harm in looting one or seven in the meantime. Store in the fridge for up to 1 month.

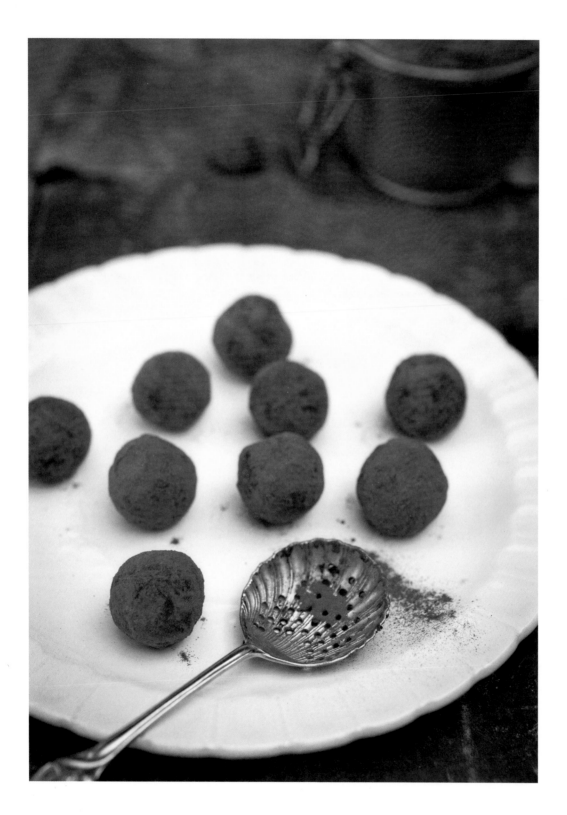

FIG AND PRUNE CRUMBLE WITH GINGER-LACED YOGURT AND DATE SYRUP

>>

This crumble will unleash some serious goodness into your system and prompt a fervent tail-wagging session around the kitchen table.

Whether fresh or dried, figs are a surprisingly good source of calcium. This mineral is the Holy Grail for strong bones, so throw a packet of dried figs in your office drawer to ward off sugar cravings and dodgy hips.

It's worth keeping your health antennae out for cold-pressed extra virgin coconut oil. Once refined, coconut oil's immune-boosting properties substantially diminish. I should add that there is quite a price difference. A large jar of copra, the refined coconut oil that you don't want, is available for the same price as a big bar of chocolate. The equivalent size, raw and unrefined, will be four times more costly. But as Michael Pollan so sensibly exhorts, "It's better to pay the grocer than the doctor."

For the filling:
6 small or medium apples
1 tablespoon ground cinnamon
Splash of lemon juice
6 fresh or dried figs, roughly chopped
Roughly 1 cup (180 g) prunes, stones removed and chopped

For the topping:
2 cups (180 g) jumbo oat flakes
4–5 tablespoons maple or brown rice syrup, honey, or raw agave nectar
4 tablespoons extra virgin coconut oil
1 cup (120 g) mixed seeds (sunflower, flaxseeds, pumpkin)
Sprinkle of sea salt flakes

For the yogurt:
Coconut or organic soy yogurt
3 tablespoons grated frozen ginger
Date syrup, to serve

Serves 8

Preheat the oven to 340°F (170°C).

To make the topping, briefly blitz the oats with the syrup and coconut oil (which is solid like butter at room temperature) in a food processor until it clumps together–5 seconds should do the trick. Stir in the seeds and salt and mix well. It's a good idea to soak the flaxseeds in twice as much water for 60 minutes or overnight, but it's not essential.

To prep the fruit, chop the apples into bite-size pieces, discarding the core. Don't remove the skins, as these soften once cooked and can add terrific texture and nutrition. In a small saucepan filled with 1 inch of boiling water, add the apples, cinnamon and lemon juice. Cover and cook on medium heat until semisquishy (anywhere between 8 and 20 minutes, depending on the variety of apple used). Remember not to let it turn into mush, as it will have additional cooking time in the oven later (but if this happens, don't panic–it will still taste damn fine!). Once it's soft, add the figs and prunes. Pour the filling into an oven dish. Top with the oaty crumble and press down.

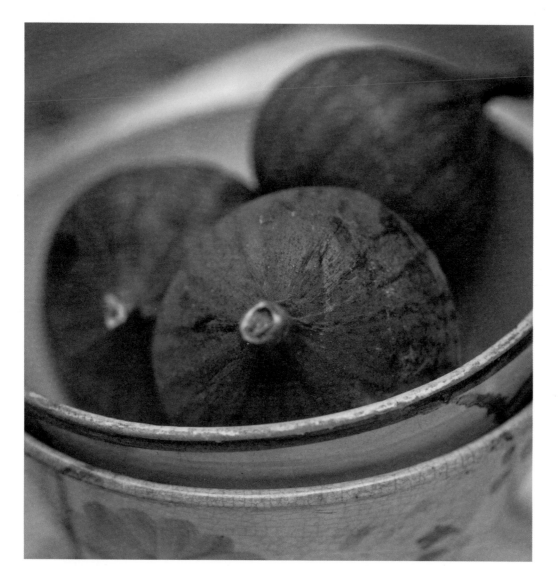

Bake for 30 minutes, making sure the top does not brown
and turn bitter. Agave will brown quickly, so you may
need to adjust the temperature if using this particular
sweetener. Allow to cool if you can overcome the
temptation to dive straight in. The crumble solidifies
when cool, but if you don't mind a crumbly crumble,
knock yourself out. Serve alongside natural yogurt laced
with frozen ginger, a bottle of date syrup, and someone
you're trying to impress.

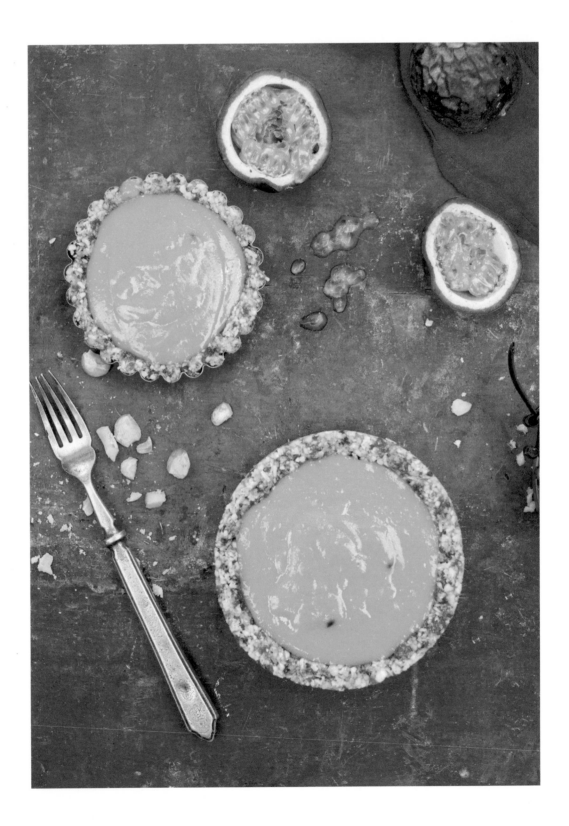

MACADAMIA AND PASSION FRUIT CUSTARD PIE

>>

This recipe will help exorcise those overactive sugar cravings. The base is both crunchy and creamy, in a way that only a team of macadamia can achieve. You'll be getting a fair whack of heart-healthy magnesium and cholesterol-lowering oleic too, something junk food could never brag.

The passion fruit filling is sweet and buttery, with a halo hovering over it. Don't be afraid of egg yolks, as they contain a brain-boosting compound called choline to help you find those bloody car keys. And while coconut oil is a source of saturated fat, its unique chemical structure allows us to utilize it as energy straightaway.

The snazziest pie dish to use is a an 8-inch loose-bottomed one, but play with whatever you have. This pie will taste sensational regardless of where you put it. Grease the base and sides with coconut oil.

Using a food processor, briefly pulse all the crust ingredients until they start to clump together in a doughy ball. Scrape into your pie dish and press along the sides and bottom with clean fingers to cover the entire dish and form a crust. If you have any mixture left over, roll into bonbons and use as bribes for stubborn toddlers and teenagers. Chill the pie crust in the freezer until later.

To make the custardy filling, first download a podcast or stick on some great tunes since you will be locked to the cooker for 8 minutes. Gently heat all the ingredients on an extra-low setting in a small saucepan. If it's too hot, the yolks will cook in seconds. Continuous whisking is crucial. When all the coconut oil has melted, keep a watch for little bubbles forming on the surface, telling you the mixture is getting hotter and hotter. By then, you should notice the mixture getting thicker, like a custard. Test it by dipping the back of a spoon into it. If the custard coats the spoon, remove it from the heat. If it runs off, keep the custard over the heat until it thickens a little more. Failure to keep whisking will result in lemony scrambled eggs.

Pour over your chilled base and set in the fridge for 2 hours before serving. Deliciously potent stuff, with a nod to the nutritional gods.

For the crust:
1 cup (140 g) raw macadamia nuts (and/or almonds)
1 cup (150 g) raisins (not currants)
$^1/_2$ cup (40 g) desiccated coconut
1 tablespoon runny honey or maple syrup

For the filling:
4 egg yolks
2 passion fruit
Juice and rind of 1 large lemon
5 tablespoons runny honey or raw agave nectar
4 tablespoons extra virgin coconut oil

Makes 12-16 portions

LEMON AND PISTACHIO PIE WITH ORANGE BLOSSOM YOGURT

>>

This recipe is designed to drive your neurotransmitters wild without driving up your blood sugar levels or clogging your arteries.

But aren't nuts fattening? Not so. Nuts contain monounsaturated fat. That's the healthy one associated with lower rates of heart disease and cholesterol. Commercial candy, on the other hand, is a source of nasty fat, responsible for bumping up your bad LDL cholesterol and haunting your arteries. Please don't confuse the two fats-they behave very differently in the body. In fact, the British Medical Journal published research on Polymeal foods that, if consumed daily, would reduce the risk of cardiovascular disease by 75 percent. Dark chocolate and nuts were two of the seven foods. Glee.

For the biscuit base:
³/₄ cup (105 g) unsalted
  cashews
¹/₂ cup (70 g) shelled
  pistachios
¹/₃ cup (50 g) sultanas
Juice and zest of 1 lemon
2 tablespoons raw agave
  nectar, or maple or brown
  rice syrup
¹/₄ teaspoon unrefined salt

For the filling:
1¹/₂ cups (200 g) raw unsalted
  cashew nuts, soaked
  overnight
¹/₂ cup (125 ml) raw agave
  nectar or brown rice syrup
  (not maple)
Up to ¹/₂ cup (125 ml) melted
  extra virgin coconut oil
Juice of 1¹/₂ lemons
¹/₂ teaspoon ground turmeric

Handful of shelled
  pistachios, to decorate
Coconut or soy yogurt,
  to serve
Orange blossom water, to
  serve

Makes 12 slices

Briefly pulse the base ingredients together using a food processor. Stop the motor when the dough starts to clump together. Spread the nutty dough over the bottom of a lightly oiled 7-inch springform pan. These are a special type of baking pan usually used to make cheesecakes. Place in the freezer to chill while you get going on the filling.

Drain the cashews and discard the soaking liquid. Cream the softened cashews with the remaining filling ingredients (except the pistachios) until smooth and glossy. This should take 2 minutes in a blender or food processor. Add more turmeric if you want to achieve an even brighter glow. Too much, though, and planes will start landing on your house. Pour over your base and return to the freezer until beckoned.

Allow to thaw for 5 minutes before cutting the pie from frozen. Crush a handful of shelled pistachios with the bottom of a saucepan and tickle the top of the pie with them. Serve with thick cultured coconut or soy yogurt splashed with orange blossom water or culinary-grade orange oil. And maybe a pitcher of iced green tea on a sweltering summer's day.

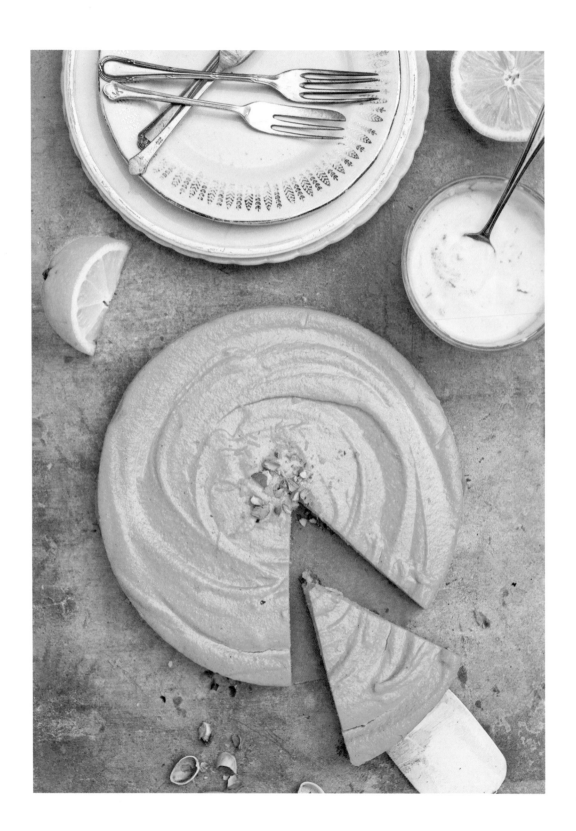

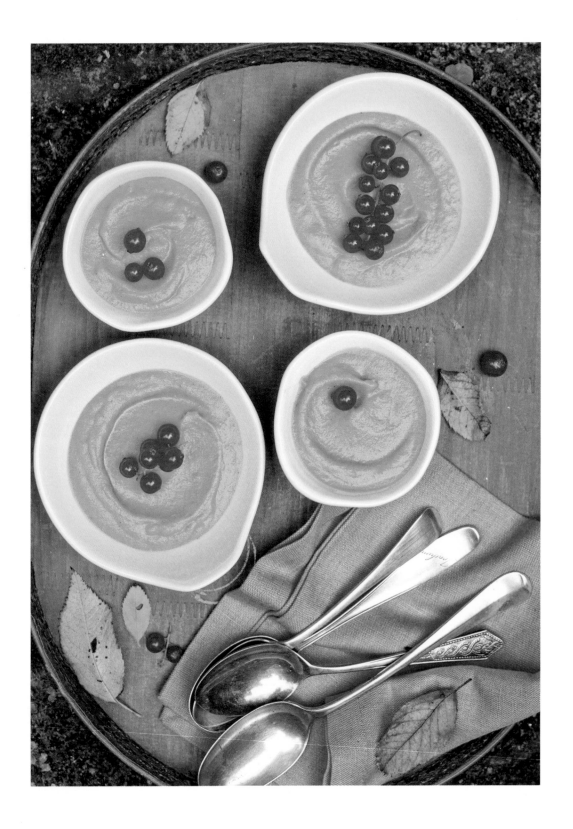

MAPLE AND PUMPKIN PANNA COTTA

>>>

The Japanese use agar as a weight-loss aid because of its stellar fiber content. This natural setting agent is made from sea algae, which is frozen and shaved. So make friends with agar, because it's good for your body. After all, you're the one who has to live in it!

Start by peeling the ginger and placing it in the freezer to firm up. Fresh ginger would be too fibrous, overpowering and stringy.

While the ginger is freezing, peel and chop your pumpkin into matchbox-sized pieces, toss in a little olive oil, season and roast on a baking tray at 400°F (200°C) for 30 minutes, until soft and tasty. Covering the tray with aluminum foil prevents any browning from occurring. Broadly speaking, it's worth cooking about 3 mugs of chopped pumpkin and gleefully gobbling up any you don't use in the recipe. As soon as the pumpkin is done, mash it while it's hot and measure out 1^1/$_2$ cups (375 ml) of the purée. Grate the frozen ginger over it using the finest part of a grater. Set aside.

Sprinkle the agar flakes into the cold water and bring to a gentle simmer for 4–5 minutes without stirring.

In the meantime, throw the remaining ingredients (except the blueberries or red currants) into your food processor along with the pumpkin mash. Blend everything together on high speed, slowly adding the hot agar mix. Purée until sumptuous and smooth.

Pour into handy jam jars ready to bring into school or work tomorrow. If serving tonight, refrigerate in a suitable large bowl or individual ramekin dishes until set. Excite with blueberries or red currants and a glorious drizzle of maple syrup.

1^1/$_2$-inch piece of fresh
  ginger, grated
1 small organic pumpkin
A little olive oil
1 tablespoon agar flakes
1 cup (250 ml) filtered water
4–5 tablespoons maple syrup,
  plus extra to serve
1–2 tablespoons extra virgin
  coconut oil
^{1}/$_4$ teaspoon sea salt flakes
Pinch of ground cinnamon
Splash of vanilla extract
Tiny squeeze of lime juice
Blueberries or red currants,
  to decorate

Serves 5–8

HAZELNUT AND RAISIN FREEZER COOKIES

>>>

It takes 4 pounds of grapes to produce a single pound of raisins. This markedly concentrates raisins' nutritional kick. Counted as one of your five a day, a handful of these chewy little candies will give you astral amounts of antioxidants and phytochemicals, equivalent to a bunch of fresh grapes. (No, not equivalent to a bottle of Merlot, but nice try. Nor does wine count as part of your five-a-day program, except in December, obviously.)

That same handful contains blushing amounts of resveratrol too, the phytonutrient that furnishes our body with anticancer infantry. Antioxidants and phytochemicals such as resveratrol are needed to deactivate menacing molecules in our bodies, more commonly referred to as free radicals. Imagine an internal Pac-Man and you've got the idea.

Now for the downsides. Research has shown that grapes carry more pesticides and agrichemicals than most other fruit. Agrichemicals don't exactly sound synonymous with good health, but the jury is still debating this one. If you're worried, the European Working Group has a handy guide to pesticide residues, downloadable online or as an app. It's a simple list of the "cleanest" fruit and veggies and the worst-offending ones for you to consult when shopping at your grocer. The president of the EWG is eager to make the case to eat more fruit and veggies, whether conventional or organic. He comes across as a smart and practical shopper rather than a loony food fascist.

With their high glycemic load, raisins are not so good for diabetics. In fact, all dried fruit carries greater glycemic indices (GI) than their fresh equivalent. This is something diabetics have to watch. Low-glycemic fruits to splurge on instead include fresh blueberries, raspberries, blackberries, red currants, black currants, and strawberries.

2 cups (200 g) ground almonds
$^1/_2$ cup (125 ml) extra virgin
  coconut oil, melted
$^1/_3$ cup (80 ml) maple syrup
$^1/_4$ cup (40 g) raisins
Handful of roasted hazelnuts,
  roughly chopped
Zest of 1 small unwaxed lemon
1 tablespoon ground ginger
$^1/_2$ teaspoon sea salt flakes

Makes 22 small cookies

Using a fork, mix everything together in a cold bowl. Grab an apricot-size piece of dough and flatten it into a cookie shape. If it's too sticky, wait until the dough has cooled and dampen your hands slightly.

Place on parchment paper and freeze-no need to cook. Once frozen, they can be stored in a freezer bag, ready to pillage at will. Other variations to play with include orange zest and cinnamon, a tablespoon of chia seeds for added omega-3 fuel, or carob powder and cacao nibs.

WHITE CACAO TRUFFLES

>>>>>>>>>>>>>>>>>>>>>>>>>>>>>

These are the stunning creation of one of Ireland's biggest food gurus, Katie Sanderson. If I won the lotto, I'd have a hotline to her kitchen.

Cacao butter may require a little savvy shopping to find. I get mine online (see page 253), where I can bulk-buy an artillery of scrumptious stuff without having to leave my lazy armchair.

Melt the cacao butter in a bain-marie. All this means is placing the broken shards of butter in a shallow bowl set over a pot of barely simmering water. Make sure the bowl is at least 4 inches above the simmering water. Remove from the heat and let the butter naturally melt over the hot water for 5 minutes.

Cream the other ingredients in a mini electric blender or food processor. Keep the motor running and slowly add the melted cacao butter in a steady stream.

Refrigerate for about 3 hours. If the mixture seems too hard or you've forgotten about it in the fridge, blitz it again to loosen it up. You might want to chill it in the food processor's bowl with the blade still in for this reason. Using a teaspoon, take a teeny amount and form a bonbon between your palms. Drop into lúcuma powder and roll again with dry fingertips. Store in the fridge until the munchies hit. Then kick your feet up and high-five Katie.

$^1/_3$ cup (80 ml) melted cacao butter

$^3/_4$ cup (200 g) hazelnut butter

$^1/_2$ cup (125 ml) raw agave, brown rice syrup or barley malt extract

3 tablespoons lúcuma powder, plus extra to dust

2 tablespoons water

1 teaspoon vanilla extract or powder

Pinch of pink Himalayan salt

Makes 40-50 truffles

PECAN PILLOWS WITH CHOCOLATE PUDDLES

>>

These are quick and easy to whip up, with remarkably few ingredients. But surely something so tasty has to be bad for you? Nope. Pecans are a rich source of zinc, the "fertility mineral" responsible for healthy hormones, radiant skin, and a Herculean immune system. These unassuming little nuts also proffer a nice dose of age-defying vitamin E, beta-sitosterol for dirty arteries, and potassium for moldy hangovers. Pecan, you is one talented nut.

The cacao bean happens to be one of nature's top sources of magnesium, the mineral associated with blood flow and good circulation. No yawning! Circulation affects the entire body, irrespective of what age you are. Think blood flow to the brain, depression, varicose veins, constipation, hypertension, erectile dysfunction, and gorgeous skin. We love you, Pecan Pillows!

1 cup (110 g) pecans
5 Medjool or other very
   sticky dates
4–5 tablespoons cocoa or
   cacao powder
2 tablespoons date, maple
   or brown rice syrup
Pinch of unrefined,
   mineral-rich salt
50 g 85% dark chocolate
1 tablespoon probiotic powder

Makes 15

Pulse the pecans, dates, cocoa, syrup, and a pinch of salt in a blender until the mix starts resembling sticky sand. Roll into 15 apricot-sized balls between the palms of your hands. Using your thumb, press a dimple into the crown of each ball. Refrigerate.

For the probiotic frosting, gently melt the chocolate over a saucepan of barely simmering water. It's easiest to use a plate that fits snugly on top of your saucepan, with only 1 inch of water beneath. As soon as the chocolate has melted, work very quickly. Remove from the heat, stir through the probiotic powder (or 1 tablespoon of yogurt will work), and immediately fill each pecan pillow with a puddle of frosting.

Try to refrigerate for 2 hours before looting. They're best hidden behind old jars of capers and gherkins at the back of the fridge. Few will find them.

STRAWBERRY SHORTBREAD

>>>>>>>>>>>>>>>>>>>>>>>>>>>>>

These chaps take a mere 3 minutes to whip up, 6 minutes to cook, and 2 seconds to devour. The cookie dough can even be eaten straight from the freezer. My mother calls them her La Prairie biscuits. In other words, a cracking antiaging brew high in vitamin E, calcium, protein, and antioxidants.

For adventurous palates, try lúcuma powder. This golden South American fruit is a scrumptious way of naturally sweetening the dough while providing niacin (vitamin B3) to fight cholesterol and depression. A toughie to find in stores, order lúcuma online or from your local health food supplier. Otherwise, stick to cheap and trusty ginger.

Preheat the oven to 340°F (170°C). Grease a baking tray.

Gently melt the coconut oil in a saucepan, then add the honey or maple syrup. Take off the heat and using a fork, combine with the remaining ingredients. Taste the mixture, ponder a little, and add more dried ginger or salt if you like.

When you're satisfied with your tasting session, mix well and form a squidgy ball of dough. Place on a piece of wax paper and press into an oblong pizza base shape about 1/4 inches deep with the base of your palm or your fingers. Cover with another sheet of wax paper, roll over it with a wine bottle to flatten it some more, then freeze for 15 minutes. This makes it easier to shape and cut into shortbread cookies, but it also ensures they don't turn into puddles in the oven.

Remove the dough from your freezer, cut out your desired shapes with a cookie cutter, and place on the greased tray. The quantity you get depends on how thin you manage to press the dough. I normally get about 30 shortbread cookies and freeze 20 of them in their raw state. Bake for approximately 5 minutes before they start to brown or color, or for 10 minutes if cooking from frozen. Allow to set on the baking tray in a cool place, out of temptation's sight. Best stored in the fridge, or in your tummy.

1/3 cup (80 ml) extra virgin coconut oil
1/2 cup (125 ml) honey or maple syrup
2 1/2 cups (250 g) ground almonds
3 tablespoons dried strawberries
2 tablespoons dried ginger or lúcuma powder
Good pinch of unrefined salt

Makes about 30 cookies

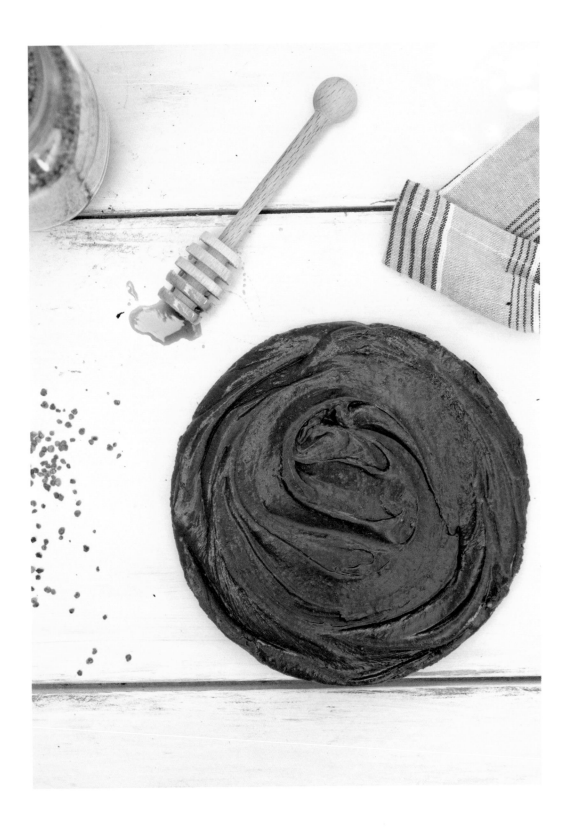

PITCH-DARK CACAO TORTE

I'm through with guilt. As a woman, my brain was trained to deliver remorseful code after every bite of chocolate cake. What if you could turn your cravings into a nutritional hit? Find something sinful but saintly? Here's a recipe for you to flirt with. It's a basic dark chocolate torte, waiting for your personalization. I decorate it with raspberry leaf tea or bee pollen, but you could try mint, ginger, sea salt, Chinese five spice, blueberry powder, or adulation.

Local unpasteurized honey is thought to help introduce manageable amounts of pollen to our bodies, allowing us to prepare for the sneezy season several months in advance. Bee pollen is another unlikely remedy for hay fever. Studies have shown how this superfood can help boost immunity and acts as a natural antihistamine. Considering the queen bee needs to lay up to 2,000 eggs per day and lives forty times longer than a worker bee, her stamina is probably testament to this luminous superfood. I think bee pollen tastes like fermented dust balls, so I've hidden it in chocolate. But I've seen people eat it straight from a jar, sober, without flinching.

Chop the dates into small pieces. Whiz in a high-speed blender with the remaining base ingredients until thoroughly socialized. You may need the teeniest splash of water to bring it together. Press the mixture firmly into a 7-inch springform circular pan. These are the funny sort of circular pans that detach from its sides. You could make a number of individual tarts too if you have a few cookie-cutter rings. Aim for a thin base. Refrigerate. Any leftover mixture? Freeze for another torte-making day or add to your morning's yogurt with blueberries and jazz.

To make the filling, cream the cashew butter, ripe avocado (if using), water, cacao, sweetener, tamari, and vanilla in a powerful blender. You should have a dense, dark, glossy ganache by now. While the motor is running, slowly add a steady stream of melted cacao butter. Taste, and decide whether you'd like more sweetness from honey or perhaps a salty kick from tamari.

Once you're happy, spread the filling over your base, decorate with bee pollen or raspberry leaf, and chill in the fridge. This torte is indecently good straight from the freezer, which is where I store mine.

For the base:
1/2 cup sticky dates, like Medjool
Up to 1 cup (120 g) walnuts
Zest of 1/2 orange
2 tablespoons carob, cacao or cocoa powder
Pinch of salt

For the filling:
1 (200 g) jar cashew butter
1/2 ripe avocado (optional)
1/4 cup (60 ml) water
5 tablespoons raw cacao or cocoa powder
4-5 tablespoons honey, or maple or date syrup
1 tablespoon tamari
1 teaspoon vanilla extract
2-3 tablespoons (45 ml) cacao butter, melted
Bee pollen granules, to decorate (optional)
1 tea bag of raspberry leaf tea, to decorate (optional)

Serves 16

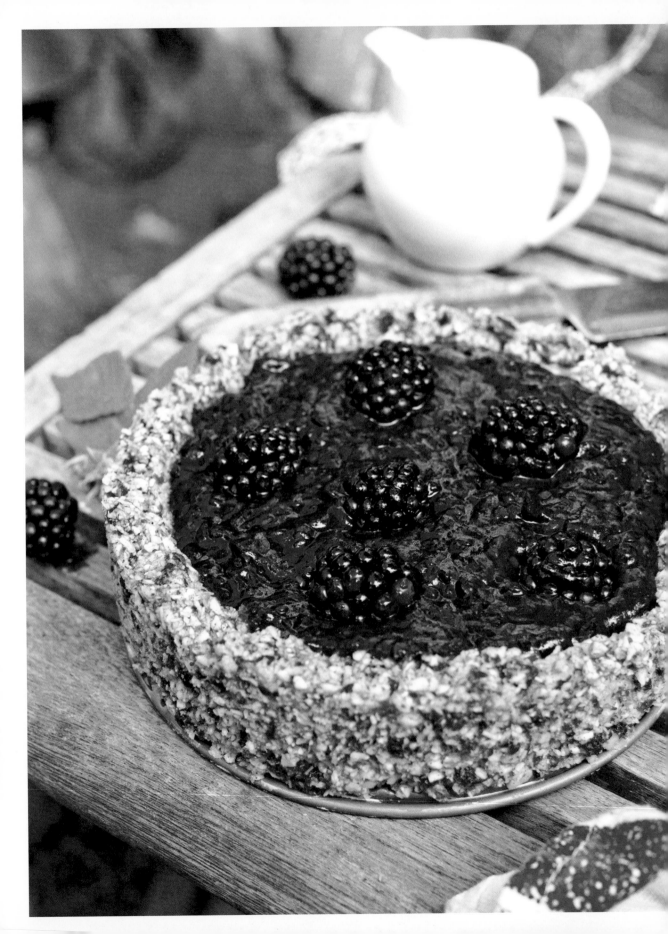

BLACKBERRY TART WITH ALMOND PASTRY

>>>

Mother Nature is preparing us for the onslaught of winter bugs by supplying us with free stashes of blackberry bushes every autumn. Blackberries are honking with vitamin C and immune-boosting carotenoids. Look up your local PYO (pick-your-own) farm instead of shooting back cold meds this autumn.

But that ain't all, my friends. This tart will arm your body with alarming amounts of antiaging artillery. This is because almonds are rich in vitamin E, the undisputed beauty vitamin, and raisins are pumped with resveratrol, a free radical assassin. Free radicals cause damage to our skin and to our bodies. Nasty things. Let's remedy that with some pie!

Using your food processor, briefly blend the pastry ingredients together until they start to clump into a doughy ball. You might need 1 teaspoon of cold water to help it along. Scrape into a pie dish and press along the sides and bottom to cover the entire dish and form a crust. Place in the freezer.

To make the jammy filling, blitz half the blackberries with all of the remaining ingredients (except the coconut yogurt) until smooth. Gently stir through the rest of the blackberries with a fork and spread over the chilled pastry. Let it set for 4 hours in the fridge and serve beside a good dollop of natural or coconut yogurt.

For the raw pastry:
1½ cups (210 g) almonds
1 cup (80 g) desiccated
  coconut
¾ cup (115 g) sultanas or
  raisins
Zest of 1 unwaxed lemon
3 tablespoons raw honey or
  maple syrup
1 teaspoon ground allspice or
  ground cinnamon
Good pinch of sea salt flakes

For the filling:
3–4 cups blackberries
8 Medjool dates
2 tablespoons raw honey or
  maple syrup (optional)
Squeeze of lemon juice
Coconut yogurt, to serve

Serves 12

POTLETS OF GRAPEFRUIT, LIME, AND GINGER CUSTARD

>>

This is a hummer of a recipe when your body feels like a petri dish. Each serving gives you more than 100 percent of your daily recommended dose of vitamin C. This is the vitamin hailed as the slayer of free radicals, active campaigner against aging, and loyal deterrent of disease. Pretty impressive for a pot of pleasure.

You'll find that freshly juiced ginger adds an extra karate kick to sore throats. Ginger is one of my top three megafoods. If you don't have a juicer at home, use your best Marilyn Monroe voice and ask your local juicing outlet to press the ginger for you. Failing this, freeze a massive 5-inch peeled stick of ginger. Grate the flesh into the mixture, straight from frozen.

6 egg yolks
Juice of 1 lime
Juice of 1 pink grapefruit
5 tablespoons extra virgin
  coconut oil
5 tablespoons raw honey
3 tablespoons juiced ginger
  (see note above)

Serves 6

Start by downloading a good podcast. You'll be locked to the stove for 8 whole minutes watching the custard thicken.

Using a small saucepan on a low setting, gently heat all the ingredients. Make sure you are continuously whisking with a metal balloon whisk. Keep a watch for little bubbles forming on the surface, telling you the mixture is getting hotter and hotter. By then you should notice it getting thicker. Test by dipping the back of a spoon into it. If the mixture coats the spoon, remove from the heat. If it runs off, keep the mixture over the heat until it thickens a little more.

Pour into little pots and refrigerate until it's no longer possible to ignore. Particularly tasty with crushed pistachio nuts or torn mint leaves.

Don't know what to do with leftover egg whites? Whip 3 into soft white peaks and add to the granola ingredients on page 20 before baking. This gives the granola extra-large clusters.

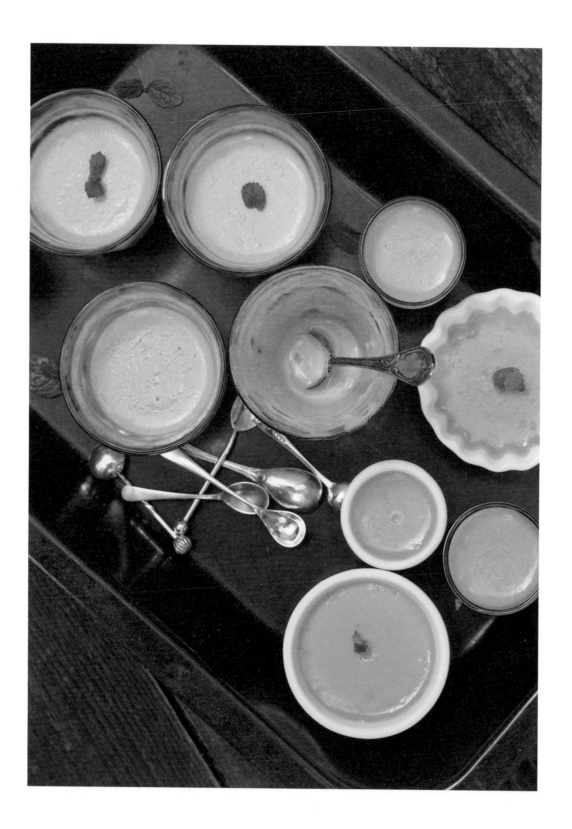

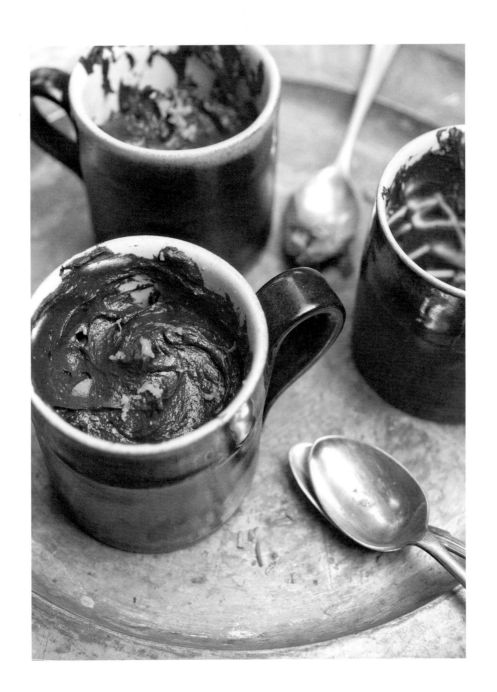

CHILI CHOCOLATE MISSILE

The addition of chili powder will give your lips a delicious sting and swell the senses. Chilies can also heighten body temperature and help release natural endorphins to keep your blood gurgling with excitement.

But wait! There's more! Folate in avocados is thought to boost histamine production, apparently necessary for optimal orgasms. Whether this is true or not, its sumptuous flesh is enough to dizzy the senses. In fact, Catholics weren't allowed to eat avocados when the Spanish conquistadors brought them back to Europe in the sixteenth century. They evoked pleasures of the flesh at a time when contraception was not available. And the Aztec people of South America-the same cunning chaps who invented hot chocolate-called the avocado plant the ahuacatl, which translates as "testicle tree."

Cream all your ingredients together with a hand-held blender. It's best chilled for 30 minutes before wolfing, but excitement may override your sensibilities. No shame in that.

Serve in petite wine glasses and top with freshly sliced red chili if you have it. This mousse is unreasonably tasty after a long day at work. You'll quickly feel the chili pelt through your veins and service those stubborn limbs.

1 ripe avocado

3 tablespoons cocoa or cacao powder

2 tablespoons raw agave nectar or maple syrup (not honey)

1 tablespoon almond, cashew, or macadamia butter

1 teaspoon tamari or a pinch of sea salt

Pinch of cayenne pepper

1 red chili, finely sliced, to decorate (optional)

Serves 2

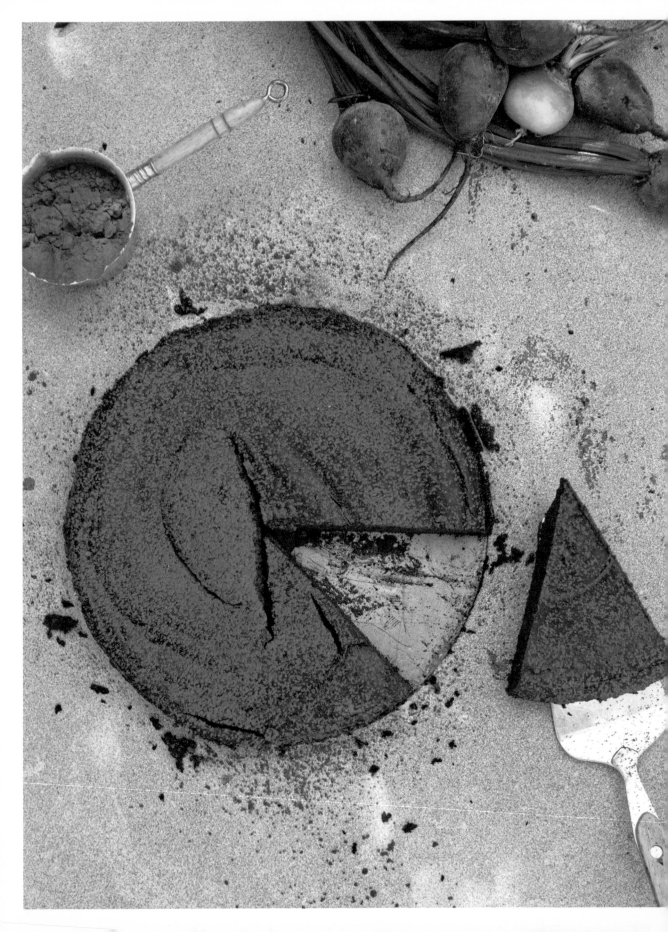

"I CAN'T BELIEVE IT'S BEETROOT" CAKE

>>>

A study in the Journal of the American Medical Association revealed that older women taking supplements might die younger than nonusers. Why? Supplements may deliver too much of a good thing, since nutrients can be toxic at high doses or over long, unsupervised periods. Or perhaps pill-poppers delegate accountability for their health to multivitamins rather than addressing their diet?

We can all agree on one thing: a diet rich in fruit, veggies, beans, and basketball will rarely backfire. I'm not saying you'll live forever (Shark Tank still has to crack that one), but we've nothing to lose by eating fresh, unadulterated food. A good diet is the best health insurance you can give your family, not a packet of lab-created pills.

I'm obsessed with beetroot right now. It's one of the tastiest vegetables on my superfood sonar. (My toddler isn't much convinced.) It may seem odd, but beetroot and chocolate are quite the couple. They get on better than Colin Farrell and Elizabeth Hurley. And the toddler is none the wiser.

Preheat the oven to 350°F (180°C). Grease an 8-inch round cake pan or springform pan.

Boil the dates in a small saucepan with about 1 inch of water for 10-15 minutes. Purée in a high-speed electric blender. This should yield about 1¹/₂ cups of date paste. The recipe needs only 1 cup's worth, so freeze the rest, use it in the Applesauce and Cinnamon Cookies on page 71, or scoff with natural yogurt.

Purée the cocoa powder, beetroot, and tamari with the date paste until sumptuously smooth. I cheat by using vacuum-packed beetroot with no vinegar.

Blend in the eggs, oil, vanilla, and baking powder until thoroughly incorporated. Immediately pour the batter into the greased cake pan.

Once the cake is in the oven, lower the heat to 340°F (170°C)-an important step. Bake for 40-55 minutes. You're looking for a moist, rich cake, not a dry, fluffy cake. It's closer to a ganache torte. Allow to cool, making sure you give it enough time to chill before removing from its pan. Serve with plenty of coconut yogurt and a large spoon.

2 cups (280 g) pitted dates
125 g cacao or cocoa powder
1 cup puréed beetroot
   (about 4 cooked baby beets
   from a vacuum packet)
2 tablespoons tamari
4 medium eggs
¹/₂ cup (125 ml) extra virgin
   olive oil
2 teaspoons vanilla extract
2 teaspoons baking powder
Natural or coconut yogurt,
   to serve (obligatory)

Serves 16-20

PRALINE CUPCAKES

>>>>>>>>>>>>>>>>>>>>>

I tend to yearn for childhood recipes, but I also love alchemizing healthier versions—coconut flour instead of refined wheat, extra virgin oils instead of butter, maple syrup instead of white sugar. Admittedly, Abba plays a big part in it too.

You can order coconut flour from your local health food store, as it's not all that common. Coconut flour is whoppingly high in fiber and low in carbohydrates, making it an ideal ingredient for celiacs, diabetics, paleos, and anyone worried about glycemic load. However, it's imperative to follow recipe measurements and not to substitute coconut flour for any other flour. It can be quite the diva.

For the cupcakes:
1/2 cup (50 g) cocoa powder
1/4 cup (35 g) coconut flour
1 teaspoon baking powder
1/2 cup (125 ml) raw agave
  nectar or honey
3 tablespoons almond butter
3 eggs, beaten
5 tablespoons melted
  coconut oil
1 tablespoon tamari
2 teaspoons apple cider
  vinegar
1 teaspoon vanilla extract

For the praline frosting:
4 tablespoons cashew butter
2-3 tablespoons maple syrup
1 teaspoon tamari
2 tablespoons melted cacao
  butter (optional)

Makes 10 cupcakes

To make the cupcakes, preheat the oven to 350°F (180°C). Sift the cocoa powder, coconut flour, and baking powder into a large mixing bowl.

In a medium bowl, beat together the agave or honey and the almond butter with a balloon whisk (those whisky-looking things you see your grandmother using to whip cream). Blend through the remaining ingredients.

Add the wet ingredients to the dry and blend thoroughly with your balloon whisk until smooth.

Prepare a 12-cup muffin tin with 10 cupcake liners and fill each one with 1/4 cup of the mixture. Expect a very runny consistency. Don't worry—you're on the right track. Bake for 20 minutes. Touch to feel if they are done. Gently remove from the muffin tin and allow to cool completely on a wire rack before icing with praline frosting.

To make the frosting, mix the nut butter, maple syrup, and tamari together with a fork. Smother on top of each cupcake and gleefully tiptoe through the kitchen. If your nut butter is fairly solid, it's a good idea to blend it with melted cacao butter to loosen it up.

Dispatches from the kitchen: You can replace the almond butter with equal amounts of soy yogurt. It seems rather important to stick to raw dark agave or honey. Maple syrup, barley malt extract, and brown rice syrup misbehave with the coconut flour.

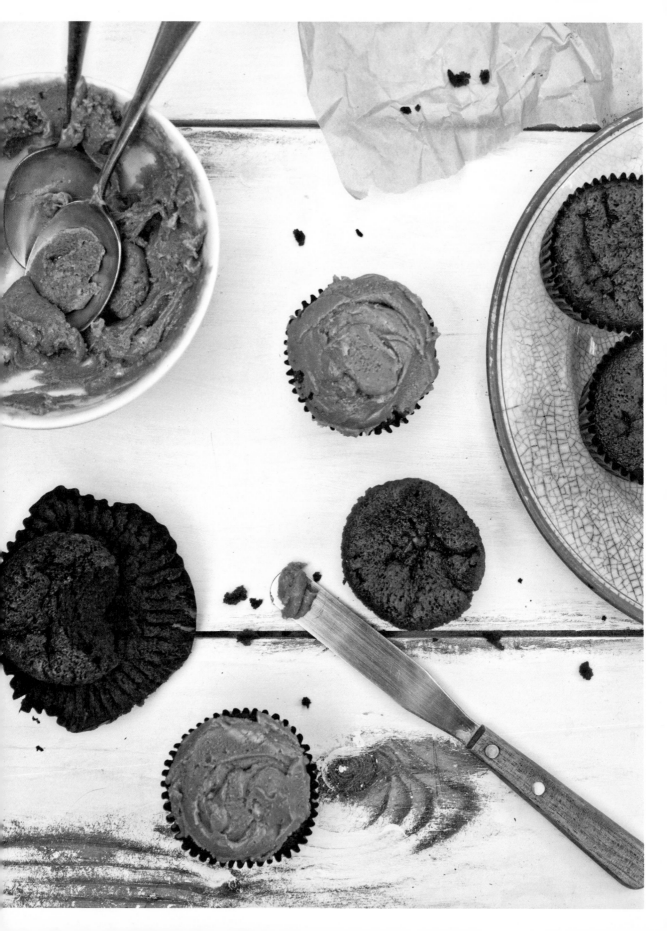

CINNAMON AND PECAN MALT ICE CREAM

>>

My husband never suspected this was dairy-free. Had I told him, perhaps his spoon would never have ventured in. It was loved, revered, and annihilated in one blissful binge.

Chilled, full-fat coconut milk is the key. Go for the organic variety; inorganic can be packed with preservatives and chemical stabilizers that turn the ice cream a dodgy tinge of purple. A top idea is to chill your serving bowls in the freezer beforehand. I use tiny glass preserving jars so that everyone has a pot to themselves.

4 frozen bananas
One 13.5 oz (398 ml) can full-
  fat coconut milk, chilled
3 tablespoons barley malt
  extract or maple syrup
¹/₂ tablespoon ground cinnamon
Handful of pecans,
  crushed, to decorate

Serves 3–4

Peel and chop each banana into many chunks. Try using black-skinned bananas, which are ultra ripe and much sweeter. Place the chunks on a breadboard covered with baking parchment, making sure the banana pieces are not touching each other. Freeze overnight, then transfer to a freezer bag. This is to prevent the banana sticking together and wearing down your food processor and your patience.

When an ice cream craving hits, take the chilled, unopened can of coconut milk from the fridge and blend in a food processor with your frozen bananas, sweetener, and cinnamon. Process in bursts at first until the bananas soften, then continuously until they develop a creamy consistency.

Decorate with crushed pecans, and more maple syrup if you fancy.

Devour immediately, and finish every last slurp because it doesn't like the freezer. Oh well.

ICED GREEN TEA AND MANUKA HONEY CUBES

>>>

When my multiple espresso regime got the heave-ho, I became possessed by the search for a worthy replacement. Decaffeinated coffee was somewhat pointless, having undergone even more chemical adulterations to remove the caffeine than Ozzy Osbourne's liver. Floral teas were cruel. I wanted a hit, not a mug of liquid lawn.

Then I tasted chilled green tea with fresh lemon. Green tea contains one-third the amount of coffee's caffeine and up to twenty times the antioxidant activity as vitamin C. This popular Chinese tea is also bucked up with skin-enhancing polyphenols, something coffee sorely envies.

Choosing to cut down on coffee is a smart decision. Coffee's giant caffeine content releases sugar into your system in the form of glycogen and makes your blood pressure pelt. That's why you love it. But your heart doesn't. Nor does your immune system, which becomes less effective under the influence of raised cortisol levels. Besides, your skin looks parched on coffee, your mouth feels like a badger's bum, and you age quicker. Onward!

Steep the bags in a teapot filled with hot water for around 30 minutes. It doesn't matter if you have a small or large teapot because you can dilute the strength with additional water afterward. Once cooled, pour into a tall glass jug and top up with filtered water to your preferred strength. I normally use 3 pints of water with 4 tea bags as a guideline. Chill in the refrigerator.

4 tea bags of white or
  green tea
Juice of 2 large lemons
4 tablespoons manuka honey

Serves 8

To make the ice, *gently* warm the lemon juice and honey together. If using manuka honey, heating too quickly destroys its potency and health-giving properties. Likewise, baking or cooking with manuka honey deletes its effectiveness against bacteria—an expensive lesson to learn. This special honey's efficacy depends on whether or not it is taken on an empty stomach, so it's ideal for this iced green tea in between meals.

Add a little water to the warm lemony mix before pouring into an ice cube tray, then freeze until set. Serve the chilled tea in its jug alongside a tall glass filled with lemony manuka ice cubes for people to help themselves. And perhaps a punnet of raspberries, or a side of last night's gossip.

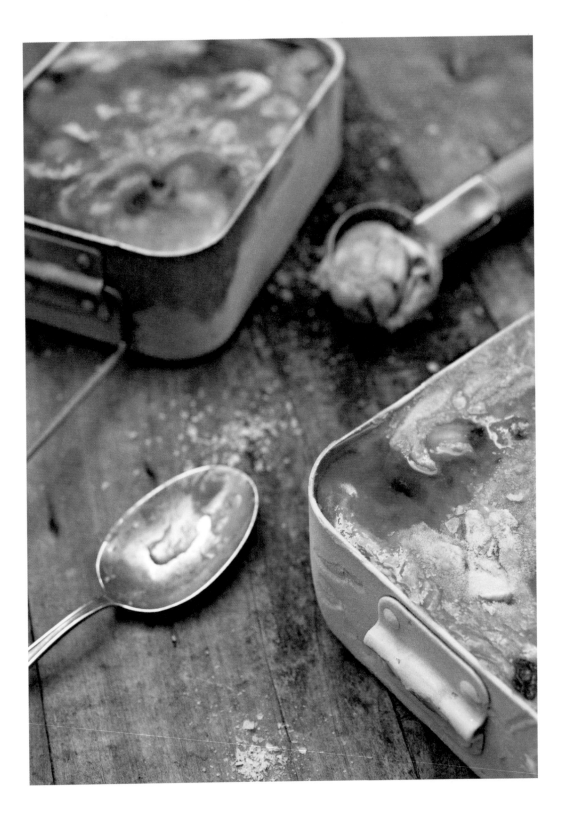

BANANA TOFFEE ICE CREAM

>>>>>>>>>>>>>>>>>>>>>>>>>>>>>>>>

Eating good food sends my hormones into party mode. It's a sensory pleasure, just like listening to great music or soaking up a swatch of unexpected sunshine. So here's my favorite ice cream recipe to feed your cells as well as your soul.

When you're looking for sweeteners, untreated honey gets my vote. Raw agave is recommended only if you suffer from wonky blood sugar levels. That's because agave has absolutely no nutritional plaudits, though it can serve as a useful alternative to sugar. For more on agave, see page 11.

Roughly mash 2¹/₂ bananas with the salt flakes. Stir through the raisins or chopped dates. I use Medjool dates because they are sent from angels. Or demons. Not sure which, but I encourage you to indulge me and try a few licky-sticky yummy ones. Dried dates are fine to use too but taste crunchy in the ice cream as opposed to squidgy. Raisins are delectably chewy and noticeably cheaper.

In a separate bowl, beat the tahini, sweetener, and vanilla with a fork until sumptuously smooth. Fold in the banana mess. Now chop the remaining 1¹/₂ bananas into chunks and stir through the entire ice cream mixture. You can swirl a little honey on top if you fancy-it sets like toffee. Scrape into a plastic cylindrical tub, seal, and freeze overnight. In the morning, you shall rejoice.

4 medium bananas
Decent pinch of sea salt flakes
Handful of plump raisins or
  chopped dates
1¹/₄ cups of tahini
¹/₂ cup (125 ml) raw honey,
  agave nectar, or maple syrup
1 teaspoon vanilla extract or
  powder
Extra honey, to decorate
  (optional)

Makes 12 servings

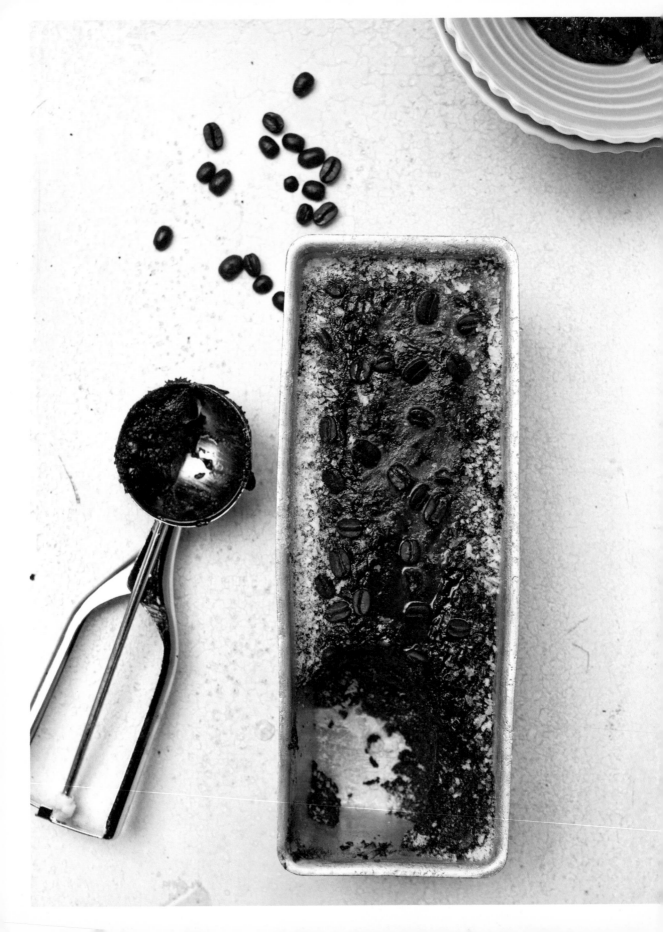

COFFEE BEAN ICE CREAM

>>>>>>>>>>>>>>>>>>>>>>>>>>>>>

In Hinduism, the sesame seed stands for immortality. Eyebrows sufficiently raised? Wait until you taste this ice cream. Notions of everlasting life will become much clearer. Theoretically, it might come from the sesame's stash of lignans. These are a group of plant-based compounds associated with fighting cancer. Or perhaps such fancy can be attributed to its bank of B vitamins? This is the vitamin responsible for releasing energy, massaging frayed nerves, and mending marriages. Not bad for half a cent per gram, and notably less than a psychotherapist.

Heat the date syrup, carob, vanilla, and salt until warm, but not burning hot.

Whisk in the tahini with a fork until sumptuously smooth. I find this a little easier if the ingredients are heated ever so gently. As you work, sprinkle in your coffee beans and good humor.

Pour the mixture into a large plastic cylindrical container, just like professional ice cream (we doubled the portions for the photo). You'll need to freeze it for 5 hours before serving.

$1^1/_4$ cups tahini
$^1/_2$ cup (125 ml) date syrup
3 tablespoons carob powder
1-2 teaspoons vanilla extract
1 teaspoon sea salt flakes
Sprinkle of whole organic
   coffee beans

Serves 6

ICE POPS

>>>>>>>>>>>>

Get yourself some fetching ice pop molds on Amazon. You could also use paper espresso cups from your local café if you ask nicely! Fill three-quarters high with ice pop mixture, cover with aluminum foil, and gently pop a wooden stick through the center of the foil. Freeze as usual. Ta-da! To-go espresso cups (as opposed to regular paper cups) are lightly lined, making it easier to remove the pop. Nifty, huh?

ISOTONIC POPS

2 cups (500 ml) young green coconut water

Pour into molds and freeze for 8 hours. That's it!

OCTONAUT ICE POPS

My little boys love The Octonauts. These cartoon sea creatures eat lots of kelp seaweed. One day, Benjamin asked me for green ice cream, just like Captain Barnacles. I couldn't resist, so here it is.

4 pears, peeled and chopped
1 small avocado
1 tablespoon wheat grass or barley grass powder

Cook the pears in a splash of water for 6-8 minutes. Keep the lid on to retain the juices. Purée with the flesh of the avocado and the wheat grass powder. You can try adding slices of kiwi too if you think your little one will eat it.

Pour into ice pop molds and freeze for 8 hours. Enough to fill 6 regular pops.

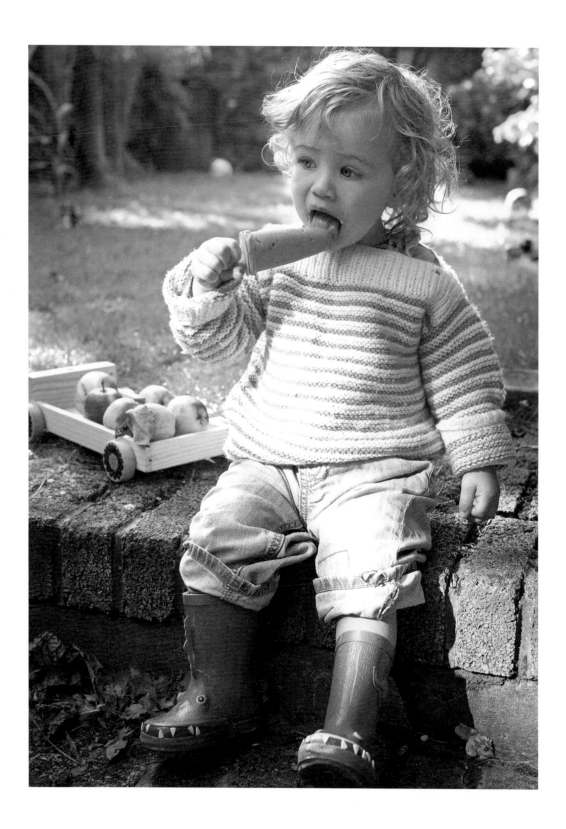

What to Read and Where to Shop

What to Read

Learning about the perils of processed food is a smart move. It's the best insurance policy you can offer your body.

My heroes are authors and campaigners like Marion Nestle, Robyn O'Brien, Joanna Blythman, Bee Wilson, Felicity Lawrence, and Michael Pollan. Never heard of them? Nestle, a professor in public health at New York University, has over 140,000 followers on Twitter. Pollan has half a million. Each of them has a free blog, so it's not necessary to shell out money to access their research and opinions. Here are some great books by these authors. Many of them read like thrillers-scandalous, jaw dropping, and haunting.

Not on the Label: What Really Goes into the Food on Your Plate by Felicity Lawrence

Eat Your Heart Out by Felicity Lawrence

Food Rules by Michael Pollan

The Food Our Children Eat by Joanna Blythman

What to Eat by Joanna Blythman

Bad Food Britain by Joanna Blythman

Swindled: From Poison Sweets to Counterfeit Coffee by Bee Wilson

The End of Overeating by David A. Kessler, M.D.

Salt Sugar Fat: How the Food Giants Hooked Us by Michael Moss

Basket Case: What's Happening to Ireland's Food? by Suzanne Campbell and Philip Boucher-Hayes

Gulp: Adventures on the Alimentary Canal by Mary Roach

Diet Delusion by Gary Taubes

Pure, White and Deadly: How Sugar Is Killing Us by Robert Lustig and John Yudkin

VB6: Eat Vegan Before 6:00 to Lose Weight and Restore Your Health. . . for Good by Mark Bittman

Good Food: Can You Trust What You Are Eating? by John McKenna

Food, Inc. (DVD) by Eric Schlosser and Robert Kenner

Farmageddon (DVD) by Linda Faillace and Kristin Canty

Where to Shop

You'll find me in quirky health stores across NYC and Dublin, organic food co-ops and specialist grocers like Whole Foods. Say hi when you see me (unless my toddler is smashing his brother's head through the deli counter again).

Some of the ingredients used throughout this book require a little detective work. I recommend exploring your nearest independent health food store, market, or savvy deli. Listed below are some useful online sources. Many deliver overseas.

www.steenbergs.co.uk
Exceptional salts and spices. Also check out the Irish Organic Herb Co. for certified organic herbs.

www.black-blum.com
Bento boxes to transport lunches to work with you.

www.amazon.com
This is where you'll find a Lurch spiralizer, nut milk bags, matcha green tea powder, oven thermometers, and specialist springform pans that I use very often.

www.avogel.ie
Three-tier large germinator or sprouter, for your bean zoo on page 126.

www.linwoodshealthfoods.com
If you don't own a coffee grinder to finely mill seeds, Linwoods does a fantastic range of freshly milled flax, sunflower, pumpkin, and chia seeds, and even goji berries. Essential for recipes such as the Flaxseed Focaccia (page 54), Office Bombs (page 62), Barley Grass Balls (page 66), and Chia Bonbons (page 64).

www.highbankorchards.com
Organic apple syrup—Ireland's answer to maple syrup.

www.blackgarlic.com
Fermented and aged black garlic. Keeps for weeks in the fridge.

www.pulsin.co.uk
For the Pea Protein Isolate Powder used in the Protein Grenades on page 69. See also www.sunwarrior.com for really good raw vegan powders.

www.bobsredmill.com
For all those fabulous new flours filling your shopping list, such as chickpea (garbanzo), brown rice flour, and sorghum. Bob's Red Mill offers everything you need for a whole-food pantry.

www.teffco.com
For online orders of teff flour, both ivory and tan. Delivered straight to your doorstep. #bodyslam

www.wholefoodsmarket.com
A phenomenal whole-foods store that stocks every single ingredient featured in this cookbook and much, much more. From quirky freeze-dried passion fruit to sprouted buckwheat granola, Whole Foods Market is a kingdom of goodness.

www.traderjoes.com
With 457 locations across the United States. Everything you need for a whole-food pantry to ensure happy pots and pans.

www.navitasnaturals.com
Where I bulk-buy raw cacao products and superfoods like lúcuma, dried mulberries, goji berries, chia, milled flax, maca, and yacón. Big fan. 100% kosher and organic.

www.frontiercoop.com
Great line of spices and baking cupboard essentials, from carob powder to nutritional yeast. Excellent ethos and top-quality produce.

www.iherb.com
All manner of superfoods, from bee pollen to cacao butter, delivered to your hands. Saves a lot of lugging and chugging, especially if you use vats of coconut oil. Use the handy search bar to find what you need. Great deals on bulk-buying, including Navitas Naturals.

www.nuts.com
Get your nut butter on. Lots of choices to stock your kitchen shelves beyond regular nuts. Bulk-buy tahini.

www.josephjoseph.com
Purveyors of groovy measuring cups. British and Australian 250-milliliter cups are important, as the American cup measures 237 milliliters. Joseph Joseph also do colorful, funky digital scales, silicone spatulas, and bowls with pouring lips for making nut milks. Free delivery to your home or office.

www.ifyoucare.com
The best baking parchment on the market. It saves on sticking and tantrums, in that order. Materials are unbleached, naturally derived, and FSC certified.

www.organicsproutedflour.net
Up your game and go for sprouted flours if your wallet permits. Sprouted flours taste slightly sweeter (score!) than regular flour, and are usually more absorbent. So I tend to use a little less flour than the recipe requires if I'm using sprouted flour.

www.massaorganics.com
Bulk-buy organic, non-gassed almonds from California.

www.coconutsecret.com
Coconut everything—coconut sugar, coconut flour, and so far, my favorite coconut nectar. Other brands can taste metallic. I use their coconut aminos as I would tamari. Coconut aminos contain considerably less salt and appeal to kids. The Snazz.

www.suzannes-specialties.com
Vegan and organic sweeteners. Really great, authentic brown rice syrup.

Index

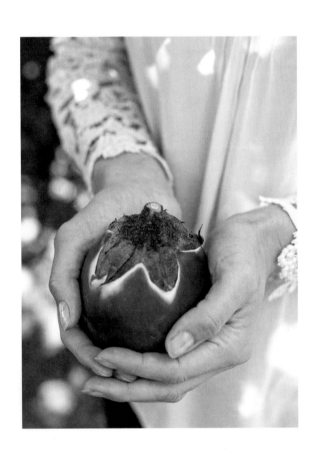